Classified Terminally Ill:
My Story of Beating the Odds

Craig V. Abbott II

&

Joseph V. Abbate, Jr.

Craig V. Abbott

Edited by Jim Farfaglia

DEDICATION

This book is dedicated to sick children everywhere, and the loving families that care for them.

ACKNOWLEDGMENTS

Craig V. Abbott II

First off, I would like to thank my close friend and co-author Joe. You're a terrific writer, and a great friend. Thank you for sharing your gift with me. I would like to thank everyone who has encouraged me to write this book, and also everyone who supports it.

I want to thank all of my wonderful nurses and doctors for keeping me so healthy for so long. To all of my friends and family, thank you for believing in me.

I especially want to thank my mother and sister. I would not be where I am today without either of you. Thank you for being an amazing family. I love you both!

Joseph V. Abbate, Jr.

I would like to thank everyone who has helped make this book possible. I would like to thank my friend and co-author, C.V., for including me in his journey, my parents for teaching me about love, family, hard work, and chasing your dreams, my friends for their help and inspiration along the way, and my wife and daughter for showing me the true meaning of love.

TABLE OF CONTENTS

FOREWARD

W. David Arnold, MD

When I first met Craig in 2010 it was a surprise, to say the least, to learn of his story. He came to see me in our neuromuscular clinic at The Ohio State University after seeking advice about his longstanding diagnosis of spinal muscular atrophy (SMA). During that first clinic visit, Craig and his mother discussed with me how he was initially diagnosed with SMA type 1 at 5 months of age by means of a muscle biopsy. We discussed how he was never able to sit independently or without support because of muscle weakness. It is necessary to point out that there are different severities of SMA, and SMA is commonly divided into at least three types. Craig was diagnosed with the most common and severe form, type 1. Consistent with Craig's story, infants affected with SMA type 1 develop symptoms prior to six months of age and are never able to sit independently.

What may not be obvious to those reading this, is how this situation provided me with great intrigue. Let me explain by providing a little additional information about the disease of SMA, particularly the severe form. The company line of those in the field of SMA is that life expectancy is less than 2 years for SMA type 1. Furthermore the available research suggested that the predicted probability of survival with SMA type 1 to age 20 is zero. So, I am in clinic seeing Craig, age 20 at this point, and he is in fact alive and he is strong enough to breathe independently. Of course my reaction as a physician and a scientist was to question whether the original diagnosis of SMA was correct or not. Nevertheless, I would point out is that all of his clinical symptoms and physical examination features were entirely consistent with the diagnosis of SMA, but his clinical severity was very much less than expected for his age. Craig and I discussed this discrepancy, and we decided to pursue genetic testing to get more definitive confirmation of the diagnosis which in turn confirmed SMA. At the time of Craig's original diagnosis at age 5 months, muscle biopsy, although invasive and imperfect, was one of the diagnostic tests of choice. The gene responsible for SMA was not determined until Craig was 6 years old. Now gene testing is the most efficient diagnostic tool, and muscle biopsy and other testing modalities are rarely needed for the diagnosis of SMA. Fortunately, genetic testing did provide Craig with a definitive diagnosis, and this left no mystery that Craig's experience with SMA was unique.

Since our first meeting I have progressed in my clinical and academic career and have developed specific interest in SMA. I now have a better understanding of how unique Craig's story is, much more than I realized during our first meeting. I have followed closely with Craig's progress during his journey while completing this book. Currently, I am studying the effects of the disease and investigating promising treatments in the laboratory and the clinic as part of a large team of experts in SMA at The Ohio State University and Nationwide Children's Hospital in Columbus, Ohio. Craig's story is motivating to me as a clinician and scientist as I see how this disease has impacted him, but most importantly how he has risen above SMA to impact so many people around him. The book captures his experiences and struggles with the disease but most importantly illustrates his determination to not allow SMA to limit his experience of life.

INTRODUCTION

In the game of life, some people are born with two strikes against them. I was born with three. Game over. Yeah, right. Well, just call me the game-changer, because I plan to shake things up a bit. I am changing the rules.

I refuse to die before I'm ready. I won't allow it. It's as simple as that. I don't care what happens; I'm not going anywhere.

Not yet.

I refuse to let anything take me, especially not a muscle-robbing, killer disease. I will fight it with every ounce of strength in my body. I will never surrender no matter how hard death tries to claim me, or how close it comes. And death has come very close.

Chapter One: I Die

My mother sat by my bedside, gently brushing a few locks of my hair across my forehead. Her fingers soothed me as they traced patterns across my brow, like a skater practicing a figure-8 over and over until it became second nature to them. I have never figured out where she found the patience – or the strength.

The gentle touch of her fingernails upon my soft skin felt good. I smiled up at her even though I knew that something was wrong again.

"You're gonna be fine," she whispered. A brave smile appeared on her face. She looked tired. Mom never ate. Mom never slept. She was just there – always – just like the snow and the cold and my disease.

Growing up in a town just downwind of Lake Ontario, you learn how to be tough. Winters here sometimes run six months long. This is not a place for sissies. It tests your will to survive. You had better be hearty if you plan to stay here. Once the calendar hits October, winter starts its icy attack; and by the time January comes to call, the weak are sent fleeing, looking for any place that will offer warmth and a respite from the howling winds and endless snow squalls.

This particular winter, the eighteenth of my life, had taken its toll on me, more so than usual. By February I had pneumonia again – for the hundredth time, for the thousandth time, no one knew; there were too times many to count. All I knew was that I had it again; and this time I had it bad.

My fever had nearly rendered me delirious. I had completely lost track of time. I tried to remember how long I had been sick. Had it been days? How many? I had no idea. All that I could feel was the familiar, gut-wrenching kick to the stomach, as clear and as unforgiving as the harsh winter winds that blew off Lake Ontario and iced my bedroom windows to the point where I could no longer see outside, trapping me in a prison cell – in a prison cell of a body that could not move on its own. This was the vulnerability of my fragile existence. This was the feeling of terminal illness, the feeling that was my life.

My college textbooks lay on the floor, closed and neglected and useless to me. I hadn't touched them in weeks. My nurse volleyed back and forth between my bed and my makeshift nightstand, overflowing with medicine bottles, medical equipment, and the controller to my X-Box. She was desperately trying to get me to breathe normally, but it was no use. Phlegm was building up in my chest and throat, and I could hardly say two words without clogging up and needing help again.

Grandpa blew a few breaths upon the glass in the door from my room to my wheelchair ramp outside. He took his shirtsleeve and rubbed hard, in circular motions, until some of the ice disappeared and there was enough room to see out. All that I could see from my bed was a dark sky, snow flying past, and the prison bars of the icicles that hung from roof edge almost to the ground.

Next to the window, Chu Chu and Layla, my lizards rested upon rocks that were heated from their overhead light, glowing orange and brown in their large aquarium. They lounged calm and restful in their simulated desert home. And though trapped in a glass tank with no promise of escape ever, they were less imprisoned than me, iced shut in my room, in a body that could hardly move a muscle.

The darkness of the winter day made the posters that covered my bedroom walls hard to see. Pictures of sun and surf and of things warm and beautiful seemed as hard to attain as a single breath. The

Metallica poster on the wall to my left, which stood guard over me as I slept, looked distant and out of focus. The band had turned away, except for James, who stared and wondered what was to become of his biggest fan.

Grandma walked into my room. She was wearing her coat buttoned all the way up to her neck, around which her scarf was wrapped tightly. She had a serious look on her face, which meant she was ready to get down to business.

"Did you call them yet, Starr?"

"No, Mom. Not yet. I'm not ready."

Grandma paced back and forth with impatient steps. She grabbed Grandpa by the arm and led him away, mumbling something under her breath. Mom leaned into me and kissed my cheek. Then, she said the dreaded words that I knew were coming all along.

"I'm sorry, Craig. You're not getting better. We have to get you to the hospital. I have to call 9-1-1. It's the only way. We have no choice."

Not again, I thought. *Oh God, please. Not again.*

I have nothing against hospitals. The place is filled with angels. I have nothing against doctors, nurses or medicine. If it weren't for them, I would have never made it to age eighteen. I would have died by age three, just like the experts had said right from the start. But going to the hospital meant pain and struggle, and I was tired of pain and struggle – so very tired. I yearned for a life without it, even if for just a few months. I needed a break. I didn't want to face another hospital stay, even if I knew it was the right thing to do. Still, I had no choice because I was *not* going to give up – ever.

I shut my eyes and tried to escape to my beach as my room started to fill with family. My nurse pressed my Cough Assist onto my face, hoping to clear my airway and make it easier for me to

5

breathe. The harsh machine had saved my life many times before, forcing a blast of air into my lungs and then sucking it back out. Up and down my chest expanded and contracted at the mercy of the medical apparatus. I felt like a rag doll attached to one of those air tubes that you see at a drive-through bank. Only this machine worked both ways, filling me with air and then sucking everything back out, over and over until my insides felt sore.

The faint voice of my mother in the distance comforted me for a moment. It was the only thing left to cling onto. I had faith in her. She was my savior, my strength, the blonde angel who watched over me. She had always fought hard to make sure nothing bad happened to me, at least nothing that she could control. But this was out of her control. I wondered how much longer she would last. What would happen if she got tired of the fight, too?

What if everyone did?

What if it didn't matter how many people were on your side? What if it didn't matter how many machines struggled to keep you alive? What if it didn't matter how many doctors you had or how much medicine you took? What if it was all in God's hands, like everyone had been saying all along? What would His decision be?

When would my time be up?

"Please hurry. He can hardly breathe," Mom said, putting the phone down and turning toward me.

I tried to force a smile, just as I am sure she did a zillion times to boost me when I needed it. But I couldn't. Not this time. I just watched her take charge of my life once again.

Returning to my bedside, Mom clutched my frail hand in hers and rubbed it as we waited for the ambulance to arrive. For a brief moment, I was at peace. I was surrounded by my family, my support system – my mom and stepdad, my grandma and grandpa – and we waited in silence for the rescuing sound of the ambulance's siren.

Then I noticed that my sister Cralynne wasn't there. She was the only one missing. I couldn't bear the thought of leaving without first seeing her.

"Where's Cray?" I said in a whisper of a voice that shook from weakness.

"No, honey. Don't talk. Shh…," Mom said. "Save your strength."

"Where's Cray?"

"She's not here right now. Please just relax."

I could barely get the words out, despite how hard I tried. A few words – a sentence, maybe two – and I was again clogged and unable to breathe. Then the cold mask descended upon my face and I was a machine again. The process was repeating itself with increased frequency and urgency.

Grandpa poked his head in to see how I was. He had tears in his eyes. I didn't like how he looked; a man who's faced usually glowed like Christmas 365 days a year. Grandpa was kind and strong, and had the faith of an Apostle. His positive attitude could fill a room with optimism; and now he had red eyes. I felt responsible.

"Where's Cray?" I repeated.

"Honey, please! Don't try to talk!"

"No, Mom. Cray!"

"Craig!"

Mom placed her hand firmly over my mouth, trying to stifle my words and help me conserve my energy. My eyes opened wide and I gasped.

"Oh my God, help him! Somebody help him! Don't talk. Please, don't talk. Just breathe!"

The Cough Assist descended onto my face again and I surrendered to it. I stopped trying to speak. I gave up and waited along with the others, looking to them for the strength that I needed and no longer had.

I was scared. I knew the trip out my bedroom door, down my winding wheelchair ramp and into the vehicle was going to be trickier than usual, given the frigid weather and my weak condition. It was going to be hard to negotiate the twists and turns of the wooden deck, especially with ice covering them. It was going to take time and I didn't have time. My breathing was getting worse by the minute.

"Where is that stupid ambulance?" Grandma let slip out.

"Mom!" snapped my mother as she glared back.

"He's gonna need to take his Cough Assist," Mom told my stepdad. "He can only go a few seconds without it. We better have it ready so we can plug it into the ambulance as soon as it gets here."

A rumble of activity on the street shook me into alertness. The sound of the siren grew from an echo in the distance to a shrill drone outside our house. It was time. Mom switched into high gear. She opened my bedroom door and a blast of February air hit me. I would have shivered if I could have. But all I could do was watch and wait.

"Over here! Hurry!" she yelled to the medical workers. Then she ran out into the street without putting on her coat. "You have to get him to the hospital!"

Grandma clutched a satchel to her chest, waiting for her cue to spring into action. Grandpa stood silently by the door and watched my mom as she checked out the ambulance and gave instructions.

My nurse continued the Cough Assist treatments; while my stepdad checked the wires and got ready to unplug it when the okay was given. Then Mom bolted back into my room, out of breath.

"Don't unplug him! Don't unplug him!" she yelled. "There's no outlet in the ambulance. There's no place to plug in the Cough Assist. He can't go. It's no good. We have to wait for another ambulance."

"Oh, my God, Starr!" Grandma said, "How long will that take?"

"I dunno, Mom. They radioed for another one. It's already on the way."

"Look at the boy," Grandpa added. "He's shaking. He's shaking! Put another blanket on him! And for goodness sakes, close that door!"

"Whatever you do, don't unplug him!" Mom repeated. "Keep the machine going as long as possible!"

Each desperate word that I heard dug up fears that I worked so hard burying. My life was hanging in the balance and time was running out. My mind was racing around inside a useless body. I had become a spectator to the events that would determine whether I lived or died.

I started playing out the scenarios in my head: dying in my room while help was far away, freezing to death on the way to the ambulance, or dying en route as we sped off to the hospital. It was hard to envision a positive outcome. The clock was ticking and I was fading. I could feel my energy draining from my body with each and every strained breath that I took. Soon, all I felt was scared.

My eyes were fixed on my mother as she paced around in front of me. Then, she again ran outside. The second ambulance was here. I tried harder to take a breath, but by this time I could feel my

9

insides choking me. I started coughing and gasping for air.

Mom was back now, but this time looking worse than before.

"No outlet. Again, there's no outlet! What do people do when they need electricity? We can't take him off the machine. It has to go with him! Don't anybody do anything; and for God's sake keep him on that machine!"

Mom ran outside again and I felt lost. I had no focus when she wasn't by my side.

A blur of people passed in front of me, each as helpless and useless as the one before. There was no way that I could leave the house without my Cough Assist. And it seemed like soon, even *that* would not help any more. My gasping grew harder and deeper as each passing breath became increasingly more difficult. It felt like my eyes would explode from my head as I struggled with all my might to take in some air. I could not swallow. I could not inhale. I could not exhale. At times, I could not tell if I was breathing at all. Then, my mother appeared again.

"It's here! And it has power!"

Everyone sprang into action.

"Wait, wait!" she said. "We can't take him off the machine until we know for sure it'll work. We need to test out the power source. I won't let Craig go until we are absolutely sure."

My stepdad grabbed my radio and ran out to the ambulance while everyone waited for the cue. A few minutes passed until he reappeared and gave us the thumbs-up. It was good to go. The only risk remaining was getting me from my bed into the ambulance without having the use of the machine that was keeping me alive.

They quickly devised a plan. It was precise and flawlessly choreographed, but any misstep could spell disaster. It just had to work. There were no other options.

Four emergency medical workers would bundle me up as warmly as possible so that I didn't freeze to death while traveling from my room to the street. Then they would pick me up and hold me at the door while I took my last deep breath using my Cough Assist. As soon as that happened, it would be unplugged so that it could be run into the ambulance, plugged in, and be ready to go when I arrived. The workers would be right behind, running as fast as they could while carrying me and trying not to slip on the icy wood of my wheel chair ramp.

The plan should have worked. But it didn't.

When they got me to the ambulance, the Cough Assist did not work. They could not turn it on. Something was wrong but no one could figure out what that was. The one machine that was keeping me alive was dead.

"What should we do?" asked my stepdad. "Take him back into his room and put him back on the machine?"

"No! We've got to get him to the hospital – NOW!" yelled the Emergency Medical Technician. "It's his only chance! It's too late to do anything else!"

Mom nodded immediately, despite knowing full well that the trip was risky and I could die along the way.

"Go!" she yelled.

I felt myself rise in the air as the E.M.T.'s hoisted the gurney, landing with a thud as its legs sprung back into position safely on the floor of the ambulance.

I was floating.

I was falling.

I was lost and it was cold and dark.

The rumble of the motor rocked me and the rhythmic whir of the machines echoed throughout the ambulance.

The stage lights brightened, and I could see that I was at a Metallica concert. Lars raised his drumstick high into the air and the bass drum pounded the seductive intro to "Enter Sandman." The show had begun.

The music called to me. I wanted to follow it.

The ambulance sped off toward the hospital. I struggled to breathe; but again could not. All I could feel inside was a horrible sense of panic as I started to choke to death on my own phlegm. As I sank deeper and deeper into a cold, dark void, I knew what was happening.

I had never been so scared in all my life. I looked up at my mother, and with every ounce of strength that I had, I mouthed the words, "I'm dying. I'm dying…" Nothing came out.

Mom grabbed my hand tight.

"Everything is going to be fine," she said. "It's such a lovely day and we're going to the beach. You know how much you love the sand and the sky and the waves. Just think about the ocean."

I could not tell what was real anymore. The drone of the siren became notes on the guitar, drowning out the sounds of the waves as they crashed against the shore. My mother's words faded. She sounded like she was talking to me at the end of a tunnel that was getting longer and longer and longer.

My heart beat in synch with the drums as they grew louder and louder. Notes floated before me, seductively teasing me to follow. The dark words filled my ears and called me to a faraway place.

"Craig, honey, hang on. Think of the beach. Think of the beach! We'll be there soon. You can have ice cream. You can see all the pretty girls. Think of how warm it will be. Stay with me. Keep your eyes open. Try to breathe."

I thought I felt someone touching me, poking and pulling me along, taking me someplace. The EMT's continued working on me, trying to keep me alive. One was pounding on my chest, hoping to break loose the congestion. Another had placed an ambu bag over my face and was trying to manually pump breath into me. A wire had been attached to my finger. They kept track of my heart rate and my oxygen level. But all that I could think of at that point was "what's the use?"

Hold my hand, Mommy. Hold it tight. Squeeze it, Mommy. Don't let me go. Mommy, please don't let me go.

The beach was gone. The ambulance was icy cold, so very cold that it froze the sun and made it drop into the sea, crashing into a million pieces. It was swept away forever, along with the receding waves.

The ambulance swayed back and forth, first tossing me roughly and then gently rocking me. Rocking me. Taking me. Floating. It felt good. The edges of the circle closed in on me, darker and darker.

Exit light.

All I could see was the blonde woman. I didn't recognize her. Her lips were moving but nothing was coming out. All sound stopped except for the music. The drums, fierce and steady. The dark notes, soothing. The talk of sleep. Restful. Peaceful. Forever. The end of the fight. I wanted it. It was time to go.

It pulled me to it, right to the very edge, as I relaxed and let it

13

take control. People faded and became music. Everything melted until there was nothing but me. I was breathing. I could move. The crowd cheered; and the circle enveloped me.

Then she was gone. The blonde woman was gone.

Enter night.

I left my mother and entered the darkness, searching for the light that had led me to that place.

Chapter Two: Death Sentence

It took quite a while for anyone to suspect that something might be wrong with me.

On August 16, 1989 the doctors presented Craig and Starr Abbott with their first child. I weighed 7 pounds and 1 ounce, and had blonde hair and brown eyes, just like my mother. I was the picture of what my parents had hoped for, a happy and healthy, bouncing baby boy. Life was perfect.

For a good six months following my birth, the Abbott household was in a perpetual state of bliss. Unfortunately, it was built upon a foundation of denial. The signs that something was wrong were everywhere. Yet my family was either blinded by bliss, or simply refused to see them. Soon everyone would come to question why their bouncing baby boy didn't bounce.

A baby is surrounded by good feelings. People clamor to hold you, feed you, and make silly faces and noises at you. And, when surrounded by this love, if your belly is full and your diaper is empty, your life is nothing but smiles. And that's just the way it was with me. I was always content and smiling. As a result, everyone assumed that I was fine. No one noticed that I did not reach for objects much and that I had trouble holding onto anything. No one noticed that I was having trouble holding my head up. When I was in someone's arms, I did not latch onto them. Everyone just thought that I was extra-affectionate and cuddly, and I was snuggling into a person when they held me. No one realized that I was not able to hold onto them.

I spent a lot of time during those early days in something called a "Jolly Jumper," which was sort of a seat that was attached to the walls of the house in an open doorway. The Jolly Jumper would hold a baby, at the same time giving them the opportunity to jump or bounce around.

I didn't bounce. I never bounced.

When placed in the Jolly Jumper, I would sit slouched low and still, smiling and watching my mother as she went about her daily chores, barely moving my head to follow her as she walked to and fro. Mom would always smile at me, and I would smile right back; so of course she had little clue that something was wrong.

There was an inkling of concern when Mom would say something to me while out of my sight. She told me later that it puzzled her that I did not turn my head to look for her. She did not know that I didn't turn my head because I couldn't.

When Grandpa was around, circumstances were a bit different. Grandpa quickly became my best buddy, my playmate, and my favorite babysitter. Filling my life with music, he always had a song to share. He was in the church choir and singing groups: and he was always belting out uplifting songs of inspiration or pop oldies from his generation.

"Showtime, C.V.," he would say. "Loosen up those pipes. Your audience is waiting.

"Gabba blabba blah."

"He talked! He did it! He said his first word! I heard him, clear as a bell!"

"What did he say?" Mom asked.

"Sounded like 'the goat is loose'," Grandpa said. "Maybe I'm wrong. Maybe it was 'coat'."

Grandpa is an eternal optimist. Even during the most blizzardy of blizzards, he knew for sure that the sun was about to pop out at any second. And, even though he got the words wrong, I was indeed trying to speak; only I was trying to say "Am I old enough to have a cookie? In about six months, I would no doubt be asking about girls, how old you had to be to get a learner's permit, and if the ladies held it against you if you were still in diapers. That's just the way my mind works.

Little by little, people started noticing my lack of physical development. Grandma was the first to notice.

"He's not rolling over yet, Starr. By now, he should be rolling over."

"Maybe he's not ready; or maybe he just doesn't want to," Mom said.

"Nonsense. He's ready. All babies are ready. All babies need to explore. I'm concerned."

"But he's always smiling and laughing. He's fine."

"He rolls over for me," said Grandpa.

"He does?" asked Grandma.

"Well, yes, he sure does, when we play on the floor and I push him. Then he rolls over fine. You should see him go."

"That is *NOT* what I meant. I'm worried about him. He should be moving a lot more. Don't you see it?"

"He's fine, Mom. He's fine. He's fine."

"He seems fine to me, too," Grandpa agreed.

When I was six months old, my mother's concern started. I still had not done anything but smile and cuddle.

One day, my cousin Kaitlyn stopped by for a visit. Kaitlyn was almost exactly the same age as me, so Mom was able to compare us. I had been placed in my Jolly Jumper, and as usual I did nothing. I just smiled up at Mom like I always did. On the other hand, Kaitlyn was bouncing all over the place, active and going crazy.

"Kaitlyn is pretty active for her age, wouldn't you say?" Mom asked my aunt.

"No, not really. She's always been active."

"Well, she's kind of fidgety, don't you think?"

"No. She's fine. Just a normal baby."

That was the day that my mother realized there was something wrong with me. It's one thing to notice that you have a problem. It's another thing to figure out what needs to be done to solve it. Mom asked everyone for advice and got a lot of different opinions. She even had my pediatrician check me. Mom was told that I was a "lazy baby." That's all he did, place a simple label on me and that was that. To this day, that annoys me.

Lazy baby! I could almost laugh when I hear those words – either that or scream. If there's anything that I have *never* been, it's lazy. I wish that I could have been able to talk when I was at the doctor's office back then. If I could have spoken up, I could have told them how ridiculous that was. I could have told them to listen to my mother. Moms know when there is something wrong. If I could have opened their eyes, how much easier things would have been. If I just could have helped. But I couldn't.

Lazy baby? Not me! Lazy? No way. Never!

My family did not feel comfortable with the label "lazy baby," but what could they do? Friends offered advice. Still, none of them had ever seen a case like mine, so everything they said simply seemed like well-wishes. We were helpless, until one day Grandma spoke up.

My grandmother is a take-charge person. She has endless energy and is always helping people. When anyone has a problem, they come to Grandma. Her brown hair may not always be combed perfectly, but that's because it got messed up while she was hard at work. And though she may be on the short side, she has the strength of five people, maybe more.

Grandma is very religious, also like most of the people in my family, and she is devoted to her church and community. Every year around Thanksgiving and Christmas, she asks for donations of food and toys and things, just so she can feed people and give them holiday gifts. That's my favorite time of the year. The house is always a mess and filled with love.

Grandma also gives good advice.

"Starr," she said, "you need to do what's right for this baby. You can't stop if your heart tells you to keep searching for answers. You owe it to C.V. You owe it to yourself. Don't worry about what anyone else thinks. Don't worry if you have to kick down doors or step on people's toes to get the answers that you need. Just do it."

Grandma's words echoed what Mom had already been feeling.

"Starr, you know what to do. You've known it all along. Do the right thing. Don't give up. Never give up. Don't stop until you have the answers. C.V. is your baby and you have got to fight for him. Don't ever give up. Don't ever give up on your child."

Mom marched straight back to the pediatrician. This time, she was firm. This time, she was even more thorough and stubborn and meticulous in explaining my condition to the doctor. She did not

19

want to leave without a better answer. And this time the doctor was more definitive with his diagnosis. The news was not good.

Mom again told the doctor about my low activity levels and how I hardly moved at all. She told him how labeling me as a lazy baby was just plain ridiculous. She told him she needed better answers. Then she said something that made the doctor realize the seriousness of my condition. She mentioned this weird thing about me, how when I would lie on my back, my legs would stick out just a bit, making me look sort of like a frog. That was all that the doctor needed to hear.

After another examination, the doctor left the room for a while, leaving only the two of us to wait for him. He returned with the news that would destroy my family.

"Mrs. Abbott, I'm afraid that I have bad news," the doctor explained in a matter-of-fact manner. "All the symptoms that you have described are the classic signs of something known as Werdnig-Hoffman's Disease. I believe that this is what Craig has."

"What are you talking about?"

"Werdnig-Hoffman's Disease. It is also known as Spinal Muscular Atrophy, Type 1."

Mom just sat there in silence and held her perfect little boy in her arms.

"Mrs. Abbott, Craig is very ill," he said. "Craig is very, *very* ill."

Mom looked down at me and pulled me even tighter to her, knowing that when I was safe in her arms like that, nothing bad could ever happen to me. I smiled up at her.

"No," she said. "No. This can't be. This is impossible."

"Mrs. Abbott, I'm afraid...."

"No! You said he was lazy. You said it yourself. Lazy. That's all. When did this go from being lazy to being very ill? Craig is happy. He never cries. He can't be ill. Maybe you were right the first time. He'll get better. He'll be fine."

"Mrs. Abbott, Craig is *not* going to get better. Craig is – "

"No! I don't believe you. How can you be so sure? You hardly examined him. How can you know for certain? Why don't you check again? Examine him again. You'll see."

"Mrs. Abbott, everything you have told me points to this."

"But Doctor. Craig can't... I can't..."

"Listen to me, Mrs. Abbott. Please. This is serious. And this is extremely rare. In fact, I have never seen a patient with Werdnig-Hoffman's"

"Never seen one? Then how can you be so sure? Tell me. How can you be so sure? You're just guessing. Isn't there some test that will tell us for sure?"

"The symptoms are classic. Everything you have told me points to this. At first I had my doubts. That's why I said 'lazy baby.' But when you said 'frog's legs,' I knew."

"No! How can anyone be sure? No one knows anything for sure. People make mistakes. Doctors misdiagnose. Sick people get better."

"Please. You have got to face the facts here."

"Craig will be fine. My baby will be fine. He's just *got* to be fine."

21

"You have got to understand. Craig is not going to be fine. His disease is serious."

"How serious?" she asked.

"The medical books say that a child born with Werdnig-Hoffman's will be very sick their entire life and their life will be short."

"How short?"

"I really can't predict that. No one can. The books say he might live to be two years old, maybe three at the most."

"But, doctor…my baby!"

"Mrs. Abbott, you're in shock. You need to take some time…"

"Time? We don't have time. You said it yourself. My boy is dying. We can't just sit around and do nothing. "

"There's nothing that can be done. Just make him comfortable. That's all."

"But, doctor…"

"Mrs. Abbott, trust me. There's nothing. No medicine. No treatment. Nothing. "

"I don't understand. Isn't there anybody working to fix this?"

"Look, the fact is that it's not worth it. This disease strikes babies, and it kills them fast. If there were a treatment, there wouldn't be anyone to give it to. By the time they get onto a ventilator, it's too late. It's virtually impossible to do research, when all the patients die so quickly."

"How can you be so cold when babies are dying?"

"That's not fair, Mrs. Abbott."

"Fair? What is fair? Is it fair that Craig has this disease? Is it fair that no one can help him? Don't talk to me about fair."

"Please, Mrs. Abbott, there's nothing more that we can do."

"How can you say that? It's not your baby. You're just tossing him away. I won't allow it. You're just a bunch of quitters, all of you!"

"Please calm down."

"I will never calm down, not as long as there is a breath left in my body – and in his."

"Fine. But my advice to you is to make Craig comfortable in his final months and enjoy your baby while you still have him."

"That's it? That's all you've got to say?"

"And you might want to start shopping around for a pine box."

Chapter 3: Alone

My family was going through a tough time. Emotions were running high; and everyone was at their wit's end to try and find information about what was happening. This was not a happy time.

I was on the verge of having some painful medical examinations. The immediate future was going to be as bad as it ever got, unless, of course, I died. Luckily I was a baby when it all happened. I do not remember the doctors or the tests. I don't remember any pain at all. Today when someone tells me about what I had to endure, I cringe. Back then, I was just as happy as ever, smiling just to be held, smiling just to be with my mom. In that sense, I was lucky.

My mom, however, wasn't as lucky. The burden of my illness – of my life – fell upon her.

What do you do when your baby is given a death sentence? How do you fight back when everyone says that it's useless to do so? How do you care for your child when no treatment is available? And how do you say goodbye when you know it's not time? These are the questions that my mother had to deal with.

With no hard facts to go on, Mom had to try and explain to everyone about my disease. Grandma was the next one to find out.

"How do you know for sure? Did they do any tests?"

Grandma asked.

"They referred us to a specialist in Syracuse. A neurologist. We have an appointment next week," Mom said.

"So, then, the doctor might be wrong."

"He said he was pretty certain."

"Pretty certain is not enough. Just wait until you get test results, "Grandma said.

"And what then?" Mom asked. "What if the tests say the same thing?"

"Then you give it to God."

"Pray? Just sit around and pray for a miracle?" Mom asked.

"No, Starr. You don't sit around. You never sit around. You work your butt off. You do whatever it takes. You see every specialist in the world. And then you give it to God."

"And you really believe that God will answer our prayers?"

"Yes, I do."

"And what if that answer is 'No.' Doesn't God sometimes answer 'No?' What then?"

"If God wants this baby, then God will take this baby."

"Mom!"

"Have faith. God will get us through this. Give it to God."

Grandma never shed a tear. She sprang into action. She placed my name on the church's prayer list, and hundreds of people prayed for me – even people who didn't have a clue who I was. Grandpa was right by Grandma's side the whole time. Grandpa's faith is just as strong. The person who had the most difficult time was my father. He couldn't handle the news.

Mom called my father and told him to come home from work right away. She didn't tell him over the phone what had happened. She knew that it would be hard to tell people, especially my father. She knew that it would be the first of many things that would be hard to do.

As soon as my father saw the look on my mother's face, he knew something was wrong.

"What's the matter, Starr?" he asked. "Is it Craig? Is it the doctor? Is something wrong?"

"Yes," she said, "Craig is sick."

"Sick? How sick? Everybody gets sick. You didn't call me home just to say he's sick, did you?"

"No. Craig is very sick."

"Very sick? What do you mean? Didn't the doctor say he was just lazy?"

"It's more than that."

"How much more?" he asked.

"Craig has a neuro-muscular disease."

"A what?" he asked. "What kind of muscular disease? Is he weak? Does he need expensive medicine? Does he need to see specialists?"

"No. It's worse than that. He has something called Werdnig-

Hoffman's. There are no specialists."

"What in the world? How long does that last? What do you do to get better?"

"You don't get better," Mom explained.

"What the hell does that mean?"

"It means that you just die. Honey, the doctor said that Craig is terminal."

My father stormed out of the room. Eventually, the stress of dealing with the many unknowns of the disease and what it would do to his first-born son took its toll. And even though he stuck with us for a while, he soon would no longer be a part of my life.

Mom turned to me and whispered, "We'll be fine, baby. We'll be fine."

The fact that my diagnosis had not yet been confirmed by any clinical tests gave my mother something to cling to. Unfortunately, the tests the neurologist performed confirmed the original hunch of my pediatrician. My mother still was unable to accept this, and, like any time when there is doubt in her mind, she never rests until she has the answers. So she returned to my pediatrician and demanded answers. If not answers, then advice.

The doctor referred us to a different neurologist, this one practicing at Strong Memorial Hospital, in Rochester, a little over an hour's drive from where we lived. So at the tender age of six months, our journey began. The Abbott family – mother, father, and son – piled into the family car to battle the icy upstate New York winter in search of answers.

The weather was bad on the day of the appointment in Rochester. Snow had fallen overnight; and it continued through the day. Temperatures alternated above and below the freezing mark, just warm enough to melt some of the snow that fell upon the roads; and just cold enough to turn that into a slick glaze of ice. Nervousness had gotten the best of my mother, and she became physically ill. We had to pull the car over several times. My family was on edge. I am certainly glad that I can only tell you what I have been told, and that these are not memories that I carry with me. This was the blessing of being a baby at the time. This is my luck.

Preliminary examinations with the experts at Strong Memorial yielded the same results. The neurologist agreed with what everyone had been saying all along. He agreed that Spinal Muscular Atrophy-Type 1 was a good possibility. But in order to be absolutely certain, more tests would need to be done, one of which being a muscle biopsy on my upper right thigh.

Through the course of my life, I have never seen my mother unable to handle a bad situation. She is as strong as they come, even when times are bad. But as she has told me many times, if anything ever came close to causing her to "lose it," it was my muscle biopsy, because I was so young when it happened.

They took us into a room and prepared me for the exam. My mother and father were right there by my side. The most difficult part of the biopsy was that they could not put me out to do the test. I guess I was in a lot of pain and probably made a lot of noise. Mom does not like to talk about that. The only thing she told me was that she was on the verge of passing out; and that a nurse had to take her into another room to be attended to. Dad stayed right there with me until it was over.

The trip back home was every bit as bad as the trip there. Bands of lake-effect snow came barreling off Lake Ontario, making the driving nearly impossible. Even worse was the fact that everyone knew that we were helpless until the test results came in. Mom and

Dad had to just sit and wait. They could do nothing until they got them. No one had any idea how long that would take.

When the results of the biopsy finally came back, the news was not good. My parents finally had answers; but they were not the answers that they were looking for. The tests confirmed it. The doctors were right all along. The muscle biopsy indicated that I did indeed have Werdnig-Hoffman's Disease, otherwise known as Spinal Muscular Atrophy Type 1, which is the most severe of the Spinal Muscular Atrophies. There was no hope. I was terminally ill. My life was going to be a short one.

Even though they had the medical answers, about a million other questions – serious questions – remained. Where would we turn for help? Who was going to take care of me? Did any treatment even exist?

Mom has always said that these were the darkest days of her life; and that my smile was the one shining light that got her through. Soon after that, I grew sicker and sicker. It looked like the doctors were right all along. It looked like I didn't have very long to live. Still, we had no idea what was in store next.

Chapter Four: Time to Say Goodbye

Relief did not come with my final diagnosis, only a feeling of helpless frustration.

Time was our enemy. My family was in a state of shock, with no place to turn for help, and the clock was ticking. The official diagnosis – a meaningless name on a piece of paper – read "Werdnig-Hoffman's Disease. Spinal Muscular Atrophy Type 1." One question remained: now what?

Doctors did not offer advice. They had none. Neighbors did not stop by to offer words of support. They did not know what to say. My family and I were on our own, playing a waiting game, with no idea when it would end.

Our daily routine was never the same after that conclusive doctor's report. I was never left alone – ever. Everyone was afraid of what would happen if I did not have someone at my side 24 hours a day. Everyone was afraid that if they left my side to answer the phone, see who was at the door, or get a drink of water, they would come back to find me gone. My family stayed up nights watching me, keeping their eyes focused on my chest to see if it was still moving and I was still breathing, making sure that I did not choke, making sure that I had everything that I needed. Nobody slept – except me.

Slowly, people started helping out and the day-to-day burden was eased a tiny bit. Folks from church came by all the time to cook or clean or assist in any way that was needed. That's when my Aunt Debbie began sitting with me a few nights each week. When she did that, it allowed everyone to go to bed and get some sleep. But, as is the pattern of my life, these periods of calm have always been broken up by frequent bouts of illness, and a great many "close calls."

My arch enemy was pneumonia. It is my kryptonite. Pneumonia is always lurking around the corner, waiting to claim me. It was the one thing that everyone feared the most. You see, even though we can't move much because of all the problems with our muscles, for kids with Werdnig-Hoffman's, breathing is our Achilles heel. It takes muscles to be able to breathe, and when those muscles go, so do you. The other muscular issues could be dealt with as long as I had people to help me out. But respiratory problems, trouble breathing, coughing, congestion, and choking made up my long list of dangers. Those were the REAL problems!

A pattern soon emerged: feel okay for a while, get sick, see doctors, recover, get worse again, get pneumonia. Over and over the pattern was repeated until you could almost plan it out on a calendar: C.V. has been okay for two weeks, so that means next week here comes pneumonia. It was almost like being on a treadmill, caught between the respite of recovery and the blackness of death.

My life's "pattern" continued until the spring of 1991. Though my life was still hard for our family, something happened to make it a little better. On April 7th of that year, a little over a year after my diagnosis, I was blessed with a beautiful sister. My parents named her Cralynne.

Having another child was risky and many people questioned my parents' decision. Werdnig-Hoffman's is a genetic disease, so there was always a chance that any child my Mom had would also have it. But you can't always follow the percentages and do what is safe. Sometimes, you just have to take a chance. Sometimes, if you have love, you can beat any odds, any prediction, or any diagnosis. Sometimes you just have to surrender to the power of love itself.

Mom was well aware of all the extra sacrifices she would have to make to have two children. The only things that she didn't realize were how deep they would be and how soon they would take place.

Soon after she was born, Cralynne suffered some complications and wound up back in the hospital. It just so happens that exactly at the same time, I was on the "Craig gets pneumonia" part of my cycle. So, I wound up in the hospital, too. I guess you could say that Mom spent a lot of time running after us. Only in this case, it wasn't chasing after kids at home, or any of that "normal" stuff. In this case it was running back and forth from hospital room to hospital room. I guess this was just our way of keeping Mom in good shape so she could chase after us when we got better. Cralynne got better right away. I didn't. In fact, I was getting worse. Soon, they had to place me into an oxygen tent to stay alive.

One night, the doctors at the hospital told my mom that they did not think I was going to make it through this bout of pneumonia. It appeared that the end was in sight. I would not live to see my second birthday, just as the medical books has predicted. The doctor took her aside to a secluded spot and broke the news.

"Mrs. Abbott, I'm afraid it's not good. I don't think that Craig has long to live. I don't think he is going to survive the night. "

"Can I hold him, doctor?" Mom asked. "Can I hold him one last time?"

"No, Mrs. Abbott. That would be too risky."

"Too risky? You just said he didn't have much time left. You just said there was no hope. Please, Doctor, just one last time. What harm can it do? He's going to die anyway. Please let me hold my baby. Just one more time before he dies. Please give me a chance to say good bye to my baby boy."

"I'm afraid I can't, Mrs. Abbott. Hospital policy. It's a legal issue. We just can't do it. Craig needs the oxygen tent. We can't let him out. I could lose my job if I allowed it. I'm terribly sorry," he said. "Why don't you just stand outside the tent and say goodbye."

"No, no. I need to hold him. I need to touch him. Please Doctor!"

"I'm afraid I can't allow it and that's all there is to it."

The doctor returned to his other patients, leaving my mother alone. She walked back to my side. Then she turned to a man standing near her. His name was Mark, and he was a respiratory therapist. He had worked with me during many of my bouts with pneumonia. He knew me and he knew my family well. He also knew faith and compassion for suffering people.

"Mark. My baby –" Mom said. "My baby is dying."

"I'll let you do it. Don't worry, Starr." He whispered. "I'll let you hold Craig."

Mark took a big chance. He went against doctor's orders. He could have been fired – or worse. Still, he did what he felt was right. Mark felt that if I was not going to live, my mother needed to hold me, even if that meant just to say goodbye. The oxygen tent was doing nothing for me. I was failing. Mark removed me from my oxygen tent, and gave me to my mother, who rocked me in her arms and said goodbye.

"My dear, sweet Craig. Mommy's here. Mommy's here and everything is going to be fine."

Her rocking was gentle and quiet like the hospital room. Only a few faint mechanical beeps could be heard.

"Oh, my boy. My sweet, sweet little boy," she said to me as she ran her finger across my delicate face the way she loved to do. "Mommy is here. Mommy is here."

Then she just rocked me and hummed a quiet song while Mark stood guard and gave my mother all the time she needed with me. No one really knows how long it was, but it was just long enough for her to once again give me life. And it was my turn to give my mother the gift of hope.

I did not die. Instead, I grew stronger. Mark put me back in the oxygen tent where I recovered. Although my mother held me to say goodbye, that never happened. After a while, my pneumonia cleared up. I guess I just needed my mother's touch.

And as for Mark, the one person who ignored the orders in favor of love and of faith, he continued his successful stay at the hospital. He also went on to become a great family friend, and my first nurse, working his special ways of helping others right in my home.

Chapter Five: Legacy

I had survived my first brush with death and it made me stronger. People have told me that, even back then, I was a fighter. Still, beating death once did not change my diagnosis. It did not mean that a long life was ahead of me. On the contrary, what it meant was that we had better prepare ourselves for the inevitable.

My family arranged for me to have around the clock nursing care, seven days a week. It was the only way the hospital would allow me to be released. It was the only way to insure my safety and well-being, no matter how fragile. Once back home and stable, my family settled into a period of relative calm.

That's when Mom started getting big ideas.

"I want to build a playground for my baby," Mom told Grandma and Grandpa.

"Oh, Honey," Grandma consoled, "I understand your frustration. But won't that only make it worse?"

"What do you mean? What could be worse? How can anything be worse than what's going to happen to my baby?"

"Don't you see, Starr? Just think about it. If Craig ever gets well enough to go to the playground, won't it be cruel to have him sit there and watch the other kids? Won't that break your heart even more to see his pain?"

"No, Mom, it won't. That's not how it will be. I'll make sure of it."

"But you've already got so much on your plate right now. Where will you find the time?"

"I will. I just will. I have to do this."

"I don't know, Starr," added Grandpa. "It sounds kind of crazy."

"It's not crazy, Dad. Anyhow, when did this family ever let a crazy idea stop them? Never."

"I know. But I want you to think about this project before you tackle it," he said.

"I have thought about it – a lot. All those endless nights watching my baby's chest, wondering if each breath was the last one. No time to sleep. Only time to worry, and to think and think and think."

"Oh, I know what you mean."

"No, you don't. No one does. Only someone who has lost a baby, only someone who will lose their baby, only they can understand."

"But shouldn't you spend your time with Craig? Shouldn't you be together for whatever time he has left?"

"I will, Mom. I always will. But I can't just sit here and wait for

38

him to die. There has to be more."

"Okay, so what about this park idea?" asked Grandpa.

Mom explained how she wanted to leave a legacy for me. She felt that a place where healthy boys and girls with good, strong muscles could run around and have fun would be a nice way to remember me and what I could not do. Mom also felt that the playground should be adapted to kids who could not do those things. She envisioned a wheelchair swing for kids who were unable to swing any other way.

"Starr," Grandma said, "I like the idea. No. I love the idea. But how will we ever pull this off? It just seems like too big a job, even for this family."

"But, Starr, I wouldn't know where to start or what to do," Grandpa added. "We could never pay for this. And where would it be? Where would we find the land?"

"If it's meant to happen, Dad, it will happen."

"I know, but just think for a minute. Think how complicated this is going to be. We'll have to go to the city. All that red tape and paperwork – and that's only if they say 'yes' in the first place. Just think of all the work. Just think of… This is going to kill us."

"Kill us? Did Craig's disease kill us? Did the doctors kill us? Did everything we went through so far kill us? How can anything be any worse than that? Kill us? I don't think so. The only thing that's gonna kill anyone is the disease. And that is gonna kill Craig. We owe it to him, Dad. We owe him this much."

"But, Honey," Grandma added. "What if…what if.."

"What if what, Mom? What if Craig dies like the doctors said?"

"Yes. What if he dies before it's done? He would never see it."

"Oh, he'll see it, alright, even if that happens. Somehow my baby will see his playground."

Grandma and Grandpa knew that my Mom had made up her mind. And Mom knew that once she had convinced them to come on board, she would have an endless supply of help. The question that remained was: how in the world do you go about building a playground? The answer was simple: hard work and determination, but doing so was not so easy.

The first step was to spread the word because we had no way of knowing what to do. We needed lots of people and lots of ideas. We didn't know how much money it would take, but we knew it would be a lot. Some people estimated that it would cost at least $50,000 to get the job done. It was obvious that we couldn't do this alone. Everyone knew that if we had a huge team of workers on our side, it would make the chances for success that much better. Reaction to the idea was mixed and varied from being skeptical to that of being overjoyed. We decided to ignore the skeptical and spend our time with the positive thinkers. That's the way my family does things.

A few blocks from our house there was a tiny park that not many people used as it had grown rundown and unsafe over the years. Our plan was to use that park – and expand it – as the ground upon which the new, memorial park was built. It would need new equipment and landscaping, but at least the land was there. My family next went to a City of Fulton Common Council meeting and presented our proposal. Their reaction was positive, and they agreed to turn over the land. We were underway. Now all we needed was money…and supplies…and construction workers.

My family had some experience fundraising for our church. Grandma had led up food drives to feed families at the holidays,

Christmas gift drives to get toys and clothes to the needy, and campaigns to raise funds for community charities, but nothing on this level. We needed a lot of help – and fast. Mom admitted to me that she put a lot of pressure on herself to get the playground built before I died. That thought is what drove her to work so hard, and to push others to keep up with her.

Soon after we were given use of the property, a news story appeared in the local papers. That is what really got things started. The town of Fulton "adopted" me and the dream of a memorial playground so that it became a city-wide effort. My face was plastered all over town. Dozens upon dozens of donation jars were made, each one had one of my baby pictures on it along with a short explanation of what we were doing. These jars were placed in local stores, businesses, restaurants – any place that would say "yes." T-shirts were made up that people could wear to help spread the word. I became a celebrity, but at a terrible cost to my family. The strain of this project almost became too much for them.

Grandma and Grandpa were always tired. Our phone was always ringing off the hook with people calling with questions or offering help in one way or another. I don't know how they held it together, but they did. My mother was beyond tired. She was becoming ill.

"Starr, we're worried about you," Grandpa explained one day after she had made her rounds to raise sponsors.

"I'm fine, Dad."

"I don't think so," Grandma added. "You never rest. Everyone needs to rest"

"I rest. I sleep."

"Rest and sleep aren't the same things," Grandma continued.

41

"You need a break from this project. Just go out and do something – for yourself."

"No, Mom, I can't."

"Starr, you can't be Superwoman. You can't. Nobody can. It's not healthy."

"Please just take a break," Grandpa pleaded.

"No. There's too much to do and no time. We don't have enough money to start construction. I have no clue how long this is going to take and I want this park built so my baby can use it. We don't have time."

"Is this his dream or yours?" Grandpa asked.

"It's everyone's dream, Dad. This needs to be done for everyone."

"But, Starr, it will never get done unless you take care of yourself," said Grandma.

"It will get done, Mom. It *will* get done."

"We don't want two funerals, Starr," said Grandma.

"God forbid!" said Grandpa.

"There won't be *any* funerals, Mom, and don't ever even think that word! God is not going to take me or my baby – not yet."

God didn't take anyone. We kept right on going. Week after week, new fundraisers were held. Nothing was too small. We sold Rice Krispy treats at the Fulton Speedway every Saturday. Popular local musician Benny Mardones held a live concert for me at Nestle Park. Sports teams donated items and they were auctioned off. People who didn't even know me held chicken barbecues and other fundraisers.

A large sign was built in town so that everyone could track how much money was raised. It was a picture of a dinosaur and dubbed the "Parkasaurus." It took many months, but we eventually had enough money to start construction. It just goes to show you how a lot of little things can add up to achieving something big: we raised $76,000!

It took almost a whole year between the time my mother got the idea to build the playground until it was completed. By the time I was two years old, the playground finally was finished. Since it was built in my honor, the playground was called C.V. Abbott Playground at Hulett Park. A big sign was put up to welcome everyone to the park. My legacy was complete. And, my mother's dream did come true. The park did have a swing that kids confined to wheelchairs could use.

The negative people were wrong. The park did get built; and I eventually did get to ride on the wheelchair swing, though that was still a while in the future. Still, I do remember the day I took my first ride as fresh and as clear as if it was only last week. It was a big day for me. My whole family was there as they moved me into position and got me ready for my very first ride ever. Everyone was smiling, but no one more than me. Every once in a while I could see someone wipe away a tear. At the time I didn't know why, but now I realize what was going through their heads. They were happy for me, but they knew that memorial playgrounds were not built for those who were alive. That was something that none of us could escape no matter how high they pushed me on my swing. The thought that I would be gone was always there.

Today I can look back to that day and see only the positive side. That was some day for sure. That was when I first realized that impossible things were possible.

Chapter Six: Home is Where the Heart Is

For people with a serious disease or illness, there comes a time in their lives when they arrive at a crossroad. At this point, you can start feeling sorry for yourself and continue to question your circumstances, or surrender to your disease. When I say surrender, I do not say it in the sense that first comes to mind. I say it in the sense that you say "Okay. I am sick. I have a disease. I accept it. Now, what can I do to make it better? What can I do to have a better life?" When you get to this crossroad, your life again changes, because you have chosen between being a coward or a fighter. I have always chosen to be a fighter. It's what my family always does.

We were still sorting things out at home. I still did not have any nurses to care for me, so we relied on family members and close friends like Aunt Debbie and others from church to pitch in. I really did need 24-hour-a-day attention, so pitching in meant an awful lot of pitching, because I could not move much of anything except my head and hands – but very little.

I needed all the regular attention that a baby needs, plus a whole lot more. Of course there was the changing and bathing and feeding, but each of these had to be done in a special way. I could not support myself, so people had to learn how to hold me correctly. When I was fed, everything had to be mashed up or in very tiny bits and pieces so that there would never, ever be anything in it that could possibly choke me. Some people might wonder how we managed; but I never heard one word mentioned about that. I suppose that when you have as much love as we did, you don't look at the world that way. You block out the idea of something being a hardship. You just get right in there and do what is required.

People have said that I was a happy baby, always content, always smiling. Well, I have two theories about that. I think that each is partly correct. The first theory is that I was happy simply because I was happy. I was surrounded by loving people and it rubbed off on me. The second theory is that I wasn't fussy because, quite frankly, I couldn't be fussy. I could not kick or flail or move around like a cranky baby. I simply did not have the ability to do those things, so I appeared to be happy all the time.

So, we again made an attempt to settle into a routine, into a new way of life. To say that my mother was dealing with a lot would be an understatement. While taking care of me – a task that alone was a full-time job that would rob anyone of all their energy – she had to raise my sister while working at a job that would raise enough money to support us. Mom was also struggling with the idea that someday, perhaps someday soon, I would not be around.

Although everyone did their very best to achieve a sort of normalcy at our house, there was one thing that no one has ever been able to change or make go away. No matter what we ever did – or ever will do – there is one label that was given to me way back then that shall stick with me as long as I live, and that is the label of being "terminally ill." That is something that was and always will be impossible for me to shed, no matter what.

During the time that everyone was trying to figure out a

comfortable routine, how to cope, and how to keep me alive, things changed a lot and things changed often. I won't lie to you and say that no one ever felt tension or stress or pressure. I know how awful that time was for my family. I have heard the stories about what happened when I was a baby hundreds and hundreds of times, more and more as I grew older and became increasingly inquisitive. Whenever I heard those stories, I had to admire my family for never giving up, and for always being concerned about me and making my life better.

There was also a lot of tension between my parents, which, thankfully, I really don't remember. But I do remember that our living situation changed a few times. My parents did eventually get separated; and Mom, Cralynne, and I moved in with my grandparents. Their house was small and really couldn't handle all of us, so we tried moving out on our own. This didn't work either. Mom was in a tough spot. She had to work to support us. She had to care for Cralynne. She had to care for me, a terminally ill child. The situation was nearly impossible. She needed help. She needed advice. She needed options.

Mom listened to the words that people were sending her way. Some people suggested staying home, which really wasn't feasible. It was suggested that I live with my grandparents because of my condition and the amount of time they could spend with me. That didn't seem right. There seemed to be no answer. Everything seemed wrong.

But finally, Mom decided that the only thing to do was to do what would be best for my health, since I was the one at risk. At times like these you put your feelings on the shelf and do what has to be done. I am certain that this was the toughest decision she had to make in her entire life. She decided that I should stay with my grandparents and she and Cralynne would live elsewhere. This way I could get better care and attention. With just me in the house with my grandparents, there would be room to care for me there, no matter who would be my caregiver: my family, friends, or health workers.

Moving out would also free up a little bit of her time so that Mom could give Cralynne the love and attention she deserved as well. She knew that this was very important, since too often all the attention my medical issues overshadowed my sister. Mom never wanted any of her children to be neglected in any way, so she found the best way to balance that out. So she decided that she would move into an apartment right behind us, where she could stay extra-close.

People have asked me if I was ever angry about that decision or if I ever felt abandoned. The answer is a firm and clear "No!" I guess it might be difficult to explain, but then again so is everything in my life. You would have to be in my shoes to understand this.

Even though we all understood this tough decision, that didn't make it any easier to do. As the day of the move drew near, Mom saddened. She questioned what she was about to do. She knew deep inside that both myself and Cralynne could get better attention this way, but she worried it would tear apart the family. She also fretted about whether or not I would understand everything that was happening and why it had to be. The last evening together under one roof was painful for her.

"Craig, Sweetie," Mom said to me, as I lay in bed with my eyes half open, "Mommy has to go for a while."

I looked at her lovingly, but really could not grasp the meaning of her words. I was used to being with a lot of people. I liked that and, I was used to short absences when Mom had to work, but the only thing that I could never get used to would be if Mom wasn't there when I needed her, when times got tough. But something deep inside told me that she would never let that happen.

The hour was getting late; and Mom had to get Cralynne home and to bed, too. Still, she lingered at my bedside, holding my small hand in hers and stroking my hair as the room grew darker and darker. "Honey," she continued, "I have to go. But I want you to listen closely and remember this. I want to show you where Mommy will be."

Mom let go of my hand and pointed toward the outside.

"Do you see that place over there?" she asked. "That is where Mommy will be living. That is where Mommy and Cralynne will sleep. That is where our beds will be."

She looked closely into my eyes and they sparkled back at her. My eyes always sparkled when I heard her voice.

"And do you feel this place over here?" she asked, touching her finger to my forehead. "This is where Mommy will be whenever you get lonely or sad, or just need to think of me. This is where I will be."

I smiled even more. I loved it when she touched my head.

"And do you feel this place over here?" she asked, touching her hand to my chest. "This is where Mommy will always be so you can feel how much she loves you. This is the place that Mommy will never leave."

I didn't understand what lay ahead. But I did understand that she was going and that she loved me. I have always understood that, and I always will. My mother then laid her head next to mine for a second. Then she kissed my cheek and silently left the room.

Mom never moved too far away, and she never stopped being

my mother. Never! I saw her every single day. She has always been there when I needed her. She has never let me down. She has always been – and will always be – my mom. My love for her will always be total and absolute. She's my mom, and now she and I have different living arrangements. It's a unique set-up, but I am used to being unique. In fact, differences don't seem so different to me.

And even though she didn't live with me, my mom never missed out on anything in my life. She still made my decisions. She made sure I never missed out on anything, and I still saw her all the time, so it never felt like we didn't live together. In fact, I admire her for having the courage to do what was best for me, even if it meant missing me now and then.

My mother has been by my side every step of the way. And, as I approached the age of two, still hanging in there, I was about to start tasting freedom – and I liked the way that it tasted.

Chapter Seven: Preschool

The clock was ticking. Everyone knew this. Everyone knew exactly what the doctors had said, so as birthday number two rolled around, people started acting as if my time was up. It didn't take a math genius to figure out that, in the equation of my life, the number of days was dwindling.

One of the toughest decisions that Mom had to make at that point was if she was going to send me to preschool or not. I was old enough to go; and my condition was stable at that time. Nurses had been contracted to come into our home and help care for me. They were by my side all the time, no matter what. That took a lot of pressure off the family. Professional health care meant that everyone would have a break to rest up. Everyone could breathe easier – except for me, of course.

But Mom was still very reluctant to send me because of my weakened immune system. She had heard what the doctors had told her. She had read the reports and looked at books until she knew the disease inside-out. Mom knew how easy it was for me to get very sick. She did not want me exposed to anything that could potentially harm me. But Mom also knew that, in order to have any quality of life, you have to step out of your comfort zone, out of the safety of your protected cocoon and take some chances. So she eventually did decide to send me to preschool along with my cousin Kaitlyn. I was very happy about that, even happier than usual.

"Mom, Dad," my mom said, "I have decided to send Craig to

preschool."

"Are you sure about this, Starr?" Grandpa asked. "What about the boy's health? This is risky, you know."

"I know, Dad," Mom explained. "I know there are a million and one germs out there, each one with my baby's name on it. I know it will be taking a chance. But I owe it to him. I can't keep him cooped up forever."

"What if something happens?" Grandma asked. "It's dangerous."

"Mom, is it really any more dangerous than being home?" she asked. "To Craig, everything is dangerous. Something bad could happen anyplace at anytime, so why sit around here?"

"Have you thought this through, Starr?" Grandpa asked.

"Don't I always, Dad?"

"Are you a hundred percent sure you want to do this?" Grandma asked.

"No, Mom, I am a *thousand* percent sure…maybe more. Craig needs to go out into the world, and not just to see doctors."

Grandma and Grandpa smiled. "Well, we agree with you. We always have. We just wanted to hear it from your lips," Grandma said.

"Yeah. No doubt about it. The boy needs to get out of the house," Grandpa added. "Now the only question is: how do we swing this?"

"I think that I have the answer," Mom offered.

At this time in my life, I was too young to be driving a

wheelchair. So, they had to find another way to get me mobile. I could not simply be carried around all day. That would be dangerous, not to mention tiring. So, in order to travel around, I was put in something called a Tumble Form. A Tumble Form is a protective device that can be described as a large, over-sized, squishy stroller. It is designed to keep an infant safe when traveling. The first time I was placed in it, it felt just like sitting on an overstuffed pillow that was filled with a cloud. I clearly remember that I loved the soft, comfortable seat in the Tumble Form, but I could not stand being pushed around. I suppose that I always had the urge to do things for myself whenever possible. It just wasn't possible to do much.

It was all set. I had my Tumble Form. Mom enrolled me in preschool and made sure that my cousin Kaitlyn would be right by my side. We set up a schedule so that I would have a caregiver with me the whole time. We were good to go, so off to preschool they took me.

I can still remember preschool clearly. And when I think back to that time in my life, all I can remember is fun. I enjoyed preschool and being around lots of other kids. I must have fit in right away, as I don't remember any kind of struggles or difficulties, just non-stop fun. My favorite part of preschool was the sandbox. It just felt so wonderful to be in there and feel the soft sand against my skin. Every day they would set me in there, propped back in the corner so that I had some support, while the nurse and the teacher moved my arms and legs all over the place. It almost felt like I was moving all by myself – almost. It was a good feeling, like being in my Tumble Form or my mother's arms.

The fun didn't stop at preschool. After school ended for the day, Kaitlyn and I came home to Grandma and Grandpa's house and made some of our own fun. We had the same routine each and every day and I loved that so much. We would arrive home, have lunch, watch "Barney," one of our favorite television shows, and then take a nap. Every day the same exact thing: preschool, lunch, "Barney," nap. It was comforting to settle in to something predictable and stable, but fun.

53

Whether anyone realized it or not, Kaitlyn also became like a caregiver to me. She was my best buddy, the young person that was around me the most. To some people, the things she did might have seemed strange, but this was all part of our world, part of my world. This was my normal.

Sometimes we would play silly games that we made up. Kaitlyn especially liked our own version of "pick-up sticks" that we invented. She would rush into the kitchen and grab a handful of straws. Then, she would wrap my fingers around them as I tried to hold onto them. Of course, I did not have the strength to do this and they would tumble out and make a mess all over the floor, much to our delight. Then she would pick them all up and we would start over. We played that game for hours at a time.

Sometimes if I was out of my Tumble Form, I might slump over or topple onto my side. Kaitlyn would just rush right in and straighten me up. If my head slouched over, she would straighten that, too. I am sure that neither one of use ever thought that there was anything weird about this, nor that she was taking care of me. All we knew was that I fell over a lot, and she picked me back up. It was just something that a buddy does for another buddy.

Our routine was comfortable and fun, but sometimes the routine got interrupted. That wasn't fun. I would end up, sooner or later, picking up a germ or succumbing to the cold weather. Unfortunately, hospitals, as well as home and preschool, were still a part of my routine.

One time, while still in preschool, I got sick and had to go back to the hospital. Since by that time we knew what to do and how to do it, we didn't worry about the circumstances. We only worried about the outcome. The time bomb of my death sentence was still ticking loud and clear. Another bout with pneumonia was no surprise. What was a surprise, however, is what a social worker at the hospital suggested to my mother.

"Mrs. Abbott," she asked, "Have you ever thought about contacting the people from the Make-A-Wish Foundation. You have heard of them, haven't you?"

"Yes," Mom replied, "I just never gave it a thought. It never entered my mind, to be honest."

"You know that the Make-A-Wish people are in the business of granting wishes to children with life-threatening illnesses."

"Yes, and I think that's wonderful," Mom said.

"Mrs. Abbott, my records show that Craig has Spinal Muscular Atrophy."

"Yes, he does."

"And what do the doctors say? What is the prognosis for him in terms of how long he will live?"

"Two to three years if we are lucky. But Craig is…"

"And how old is Craig now?"

"Just about two and a half," Mom answered.

"Well? What are you waiting for? I am sure that you are well-aware that time may be running out. Why don't you give it a shot? I can put you in touch with them. I think you have a good chance."

"Well…I don't know. It seems like a big step. Right now, Craig is…"

"Really? What are you waiting for, Mrs. Abbott? What's stopping you?"

Mom thought for a second. Then she realized what she had to do. She got in touch with the people at the Make-A-Wish

Foundation and they told her that since I was terminal, I did qualify and that they would make my dream come true. The next step was for Mom to find out what my dream was.

It's funny when you start talking about dreams and having them come true. It's also kind of funny how dreams can change depending upon how old you are and where you are in your life. I am sure that if you asked Mom about what her dream would be, she would have picked having my disease cured. If you had asked me when I was a little older, I probably would have asked for the same thing, but not for myself. I would have wanted it so that the people in my life did not have to struggle so much in taking care of me. But they didn't ask me the question when I was old enough to think like that. They asked me the question when I was a little kid, so I answered the way that a little kid would.

Lots of ideas went through my head. When someone tells you that they will make any wish come true, well, that's even better than Christmas. On Christmas, you can only hope that Santa will bring you something from off of your list. This was different. This was a sure thing.

My mind got cloudy. I pictured spending a week with Barney. I pictured spending a week in an ice cream factory. Then I pictured doing both at the same time. It was clear that I was having a tough time thinking straight. Too much pressure. Then a vision came into my head. It was a commercial that I had seen on television – a commercial about a magic place where every dream came true. So, I blurted it out and that was that.

I told my Mom that my dream was to go to Disney World. Sure enough, my dream came true.

Now if you ask me a lot of specific questions about the trip, I would have to be honest and say that I don't remember many of the details. But there are some things that I do. For one thing, I do remember having a lot of fun. I can remember being in my Tumble Form and going all over the place and feeling even happier than

56

when I was at preschool. But the biggest thing that I remember is that the whole family went on this vacation together: me, Cralynne, Grandma, Grandpa, Mom, and even my father. I think that was the last time we ever did anything together.

Chapter Eight: Going Mobile

It was the single happiest day of my life so far, a wonderful memory that I carry with me to this day; but I am sure that if you ask my family, they might tell you a different story.

I can still remember the first time that they put me into it. I didn't like the way that it felt. It was big. It was scary. Even so, I was psyched. This was my first wheelchair.

My Tumble Form was all soft and squishy, just like a pillowy bed, good for sleeping in, good for taking with you for a night on the town. But the wheelchair felt different. It was large, cold and clumsy. It had gadgets all over the place. It didn't feel so warm and friendly at first. It felt like another medical device. It reminded me more of my trips to the hospital. At first, I wasn't sure if I wanted to sit in it or not; not until the doctor told me what it would do.

They placed me in the chair and positioned me. A big, black Velcro strap was tightened across my forehead to keep me upright and still. My head had to be put into place so that it would not move around, tilt over, or cause me any pain or discomfort. It didn't feel very good to have everyone moving me like that, not like the way the sandbox or the Tumble Form felt. Those were soft and warm, almost like being held in someone's arms. This was cold. This was uncomfortable. My arms and legs had to go into place, too. I almost felt like a prisoner, until "the warden" handed me the key to my escape:

A man placed my arm on the arm of the chair and showed me this little device that looked a lot like a joystick to a video game. That device controlled the wheelchair.

"Craig, this little stick here controls your wheelchair," he explained, as he placed my arm down upon it, allowing my fingers to grab onto it. "It's very easy to operate. If you want to move left, you just press the stick that way. If you want to go right, then press it right."

That was all that I needed to hear. As soon as he told me that, I started pushing it with all of my might. The wheelchair started up and I began to move. I almost got away from everyone. They had to take my hand off it to keep me from going crazy.

Later, Mark (the therapist I mentioned earlier) convinced my mom to take me to a shopping mall so that I could have a little test drive where there was more open space and my chances of doing any major damage was a lot less. I guess I should have told them that I had other plans. On second thought, they would not have let me loose if I had.

My family was there along with Mark who used to care for me from time to time. I guess that Mark liked to think the same way that I did. I guess that we both like to take chances and experience life. Maybe you could call us daredevils. I just think of it as having fun.

My family did not want me to touch the controller until we were inside the mall, at a place that was safe and deserted. They knew me well. They knew how much I liked motion and traveling. They knew that as soon I had the chance to become mobile I would be leaving people in my dust. They knew that even though I was just short of three years old, I had all the makings of a speed demon.

While my family watched me, half in excitement, half in trepidation, Mark wheeled me into a large department store.

"Okay, Buddy, ready to take a test spin?"

What was I going to say? No? No way! I could hardly contain myself. It's just a good thing that I didn't tell anyone my intentions or else they would have never handed the control over.

I smiled at him.

"Yeah!" I said loudly.

In hindsight, I think that Mark then did something that might not have been too wise. I found out later that my family didn't enjoy it much, but I sure did. Mark leaned over, cranked up the speed control dial to "supersonic," and said, "Okay, Buddy, take off!"

And that is exactly what I did.

In a split second I was off at breakneck speed, zooming my way through aisle after aisle, past racks of clothing, counters piled high with perfume, and mannequins wearing all sorts of colorful clothes. It was so exciting! This was for me!

I could hear my family yelling from afar and the voice of Mark as he was catching up behind me, telling me to slow down and take it easy. No way. It was too much fun.

People smiled at me as I whizzed by. That is, of course, until they heard my folks yelling at me to stop. I didn't care. Not one bit.

I pressed my hand as hard as I could against the controller

and kept right on going. I sped past the jewelry counter. I weaved a path through that store as fast as my wheels could go. That is when I exited the store and went into the main section of the mall.

I passed people of all shapes, colors and sizes, all going way too slow. A quick press to the left and I dodged one man. A press to the right, and I avoided two ladies with shopping bags. I thought about going into another store; maybe do some early Christmas shopping, but the aisles would only slow me down. I stuck to the straightaway. I needed speed.

"Stop! C.V., stop!" Mark shouted from somewhere behind me. I could tell he was out of breath and probably starting to get annoyed. I couldn't hear my family any longer, so I assumed I had lost them somewhere in my tracks, maybe back by the food court.

I kept going, passing store after store, looking for one to enter. Shoe store. Ick. Jewelry store. No way. Ladies underwear store. Nope. Soon I saw a pet store and thought, "That's for me." I headed straight for it and zoomed inside.

This was for me! Pets everywhere! Dogs, cats, fish! I managed to maneuver my way around, never hitting a single thing. I didn't knock over any displays or crash into any of the fish tanks or kill any of the people who I passed along the way.

Mark finally caught up to me. He was out of breath and looked frazzled. He removed my hand from the controller. Then he gave me a little lecture.

"Whoa, Buddy, you've got to slow down a little. You scared everyone by taking off like that. Slow down, okay?"

"No."

"Come on, C.V. you can't ride around like that or they won't put you in the chair, understand?"

I still wasn't convinced.

"I'll be lucky if they don't kill me for letting you get away like that. I'll be lucky if they let me take care of you anymore."

Finally, he made his point.

"We have got to teach you a few of the rules about how to use this thing."

By that time, the rest of my family caught up to us. They did not look happy.

Words were spoken; but I didn't hear a single one. Lectures were given; all going in one ear and out the other. Rules were laid down; but I forgot them. I had to. I wasn't going to let rules get in my way. I wasn't going to let silly rules stop me from doing what I needed to do.

That was the very first time that I could ever go anyplace without being carried or pushed, the first time I could move around all by myself, by the touch of my own hand on a tiny little lever. It was my first taste of freedom – my Independence Day.

That was the day that I got my legs!

Chapter Nine: The Outside World

Once I got my first taste of freedom, I was never the same. I was a boy who loved adventure and needed it even more. I wanted to go to more places and do more things, mainly because I could get around by myself and didn't have to rely on others as much. That is such a wonderful feeling. Once I became used to my new wheelchair, I started spending more and more time in it, and less time in my Tumble Form. This was the first major turning point in my life. I didn't know where I was headed, but I knew that I was on my way.

Another wonderful thing happened at about that same time. Although nothing had changed – not my illness, not my day-to-day health, not my diagnosis – people began to start thinking differently about me. They started forgetting I was ill and I loved it.

Until that time, people looked at me the same way they look at a baseball player who is in the middle of a hitting streak, noticing me, cheering me on, while at the same time wondering when it will come to an end. That was my life. Would it end today, or the next day, or the next? It was supposed to end soon – only it didn't. It went on past two and three and four years. Something amazing was happening. This was beyond the "miraculous" that the doctors had talked about. The doctors had said that in the remote chance I lived past the age of two, the only way I would ever be kept alive would be if I was put on a ventilator to keep me breathing. But I kept breathing all on my own.

Questions remained: How long could I keep going like this? Was the end in sight, or far, far away? What should I do until that time came? The answer was, and is an easy one: just keep going. Live life to the fullest. Don't worry about the end. No one knows when that will be. I know that it sounds cliché, but sometimes the truth is like that. You really do have to live each day like it was your last. You just have to keep going. Good things will happen. Never give up. Just keep going.

So, it became time for me to take another step forward. It was time to take the big leap and start elementary school. Despite all of my illnesses and time in the hospital, I started school right on schedule, with kids my own age. I am very proud of that. One of the reasons that I developed right alongside everyone else is due to some of the advantages I have had. Yes, I *did* say advantages. You see, the mere fact that I was always so ill meant that somebody had to be with me all the time. I was never alone. Never.

When people are with you all the time, you develop strong social skills. Someone is always talking to you, reading to you, teaching you things, and caring for you. So, you feel warm and friendly with everyone. When people are always asking you questions about how you feel or if something hurts, you learn how to speak at an early age. When doctors are always trying to explain to you what is going on, you learn a lot about getting along with other people who might be doing uncomfortable things to you. You receive this whole crash course in human behavior, all because you are dying. You really do pack a lot of living into a few, short years. Can you imagine what life would be like if we packed all that living into every year?

It was difficult to sleep the night before I started school. I must have driven everyone nuts. I just couldn't shut my eyes. I was too excited. Who can sleep when something this big is about to happen? Not me. Elementary school – wow! Hundreds of kids. Dozens and dozens of teachers. Eating in a cafeteria. At the tender age of five, I felt like a man of the world.

I kept the nurse very busy that night. Every few minutes I needed a drink of water or a snack. And of course that meant a few extra trips to the bathroom. Yes, I can be a handful when I want to be. I won't deny it.

Waking up the next morning was like waking up on Christmas morning – well, almost. Nothing can compare to Christmas, but this came pretty close. I was up at the crack of dawn, bugging my nurse to get me cleaned and dressed quickly so we could "go, go, go" as I liked to say all the time. That's when I realized that the world was not traveling at my pace.

"Shhhh," the nurse said in a whisper, "everyone is still asleep."

"Go, go, go!"

"Craig, it's 6:00 am. School doesn't start for over two hours. We have plenty of time."

"Go, go, go!"

"You've got to be quiet or you'll… Too late."

We heard the sound of Grandma shuffling around in the kitchen. The day was officially allowed to begin.

I am sure that they had a hard time feeding me that day because I just wanted to gobble everything in a hurry and get out of the house. Gobbling food has always been a strict no-no for me because of the choking danger. I certainly didn't make it easy for anyone that day.

Finally I was all set to go, my morning ritual completed. My nurse had bathed and dressed me, and my belly was full. I was all squeaky clean and shiny, smiling from ear to ear as I sat impatiently in my wheelchair and awaited being loaded into the van. If I could have bounced, I would have been bouncing off the walls. And if I could have walked, well, I would have probably already run out the door and down the street. On that day, my illness probably kept me a bit safer. At least they could keep me still and under control – for a while.

Once inside the van, I dreamt of what kindergarten would be like. Would the teacher be pretty? Would the kids become my new friends? How big was the sandbox? Did they have any pet animals in the room? This was going to be great!

But few things – even the good things in life – ever quite match the wild dreams that one gets in their head. Kindergarten was nice, but it wasn't the non-stop party that I had expected. In fact, it was kind of dull. Sure, my teacher was nice. Yes, the kids were friendly. And of course we did have fun. But there were other things, things that I had not expected. We had snack time, which was good; but the snacks had to be healthy ones. We had rules that we had to follow, which is good; but we had to sit still and behave, which is not always great when you want to "go, go, go." But the worst thing of all was nap time. I did not like to take naps. I had outgrown naps years ago.

There are certain things that stick with me from those first few years of elementary school. Some were good, others not so good. But I will say this: for every not-so-good thing, there was at least one thing to balance it out and make it positive. For example, I didn't like fire drills. I hated the surprise of the loud sudden noise. It scared me worse than the screech of the ambulance siren taking me to the hospital. To help me cope with this, the Principal's office would tell my teacher ahead of time so that I could always be ready. Problem solved. Also, we didn't have a sandbox. But we did have a large, colorful playground. That was even better because more kids could have fun at the same time. The cafeteria didn't always smell great, not like Grandma's kitchen at all. But occasionally we did get pizza, so that made up for the days when you didn't know what you were eating. I think life is just like this. There's always a way to solve your problems, always a playground just around the corner or a pizza just coming out of the oven.

One of my favorite memories from elementary school is Halloween. Granby Elementary School really did it up big time at Halloween. Each year, the whole class, and even some of the teachers and staff, would dress up in all kinds of costumes. Then we all marched in a big parade around the school. After the parade, parents were allowed to come in and bring cake and cookies for the class. My mom and grandpa usually came to the after party. I really enjoyed the Halloween party because it was almost how I had imagined school to be in the first place; only in my imagination we always had more cake.

I think that in many ways, Halloween is symbolic of life. The main difference is that on Halloween people wear their costumes on the outside. The rest of the time, they wear them inside to keep them hidden and secret. I don't like those secrets at all. On Halloween, you usually can tell that the kid in the scary costume with the eyeballs hanging out is a bad guy. In life, you can't tell this right away. That's one thing that I noticed in elementary school. Most of the kids were honest and direct with me. I liked it when a kid would stare at me and ask:

"What happened to you?" or "Are you sick?" or "Can you move anything?"

That was pure. That was honest. That was equality. That was the way that I liked things to be.

What I didn't like is when someone would turn away or stare out of the corner of their eye or avoid me. No matter what reason – pity, discomfort, whatever – it was inequality, and I could never stand for that! Soon I would have my worst encounter with inequality. It would turn out to be my single worst year of elementary school.

PICTURES

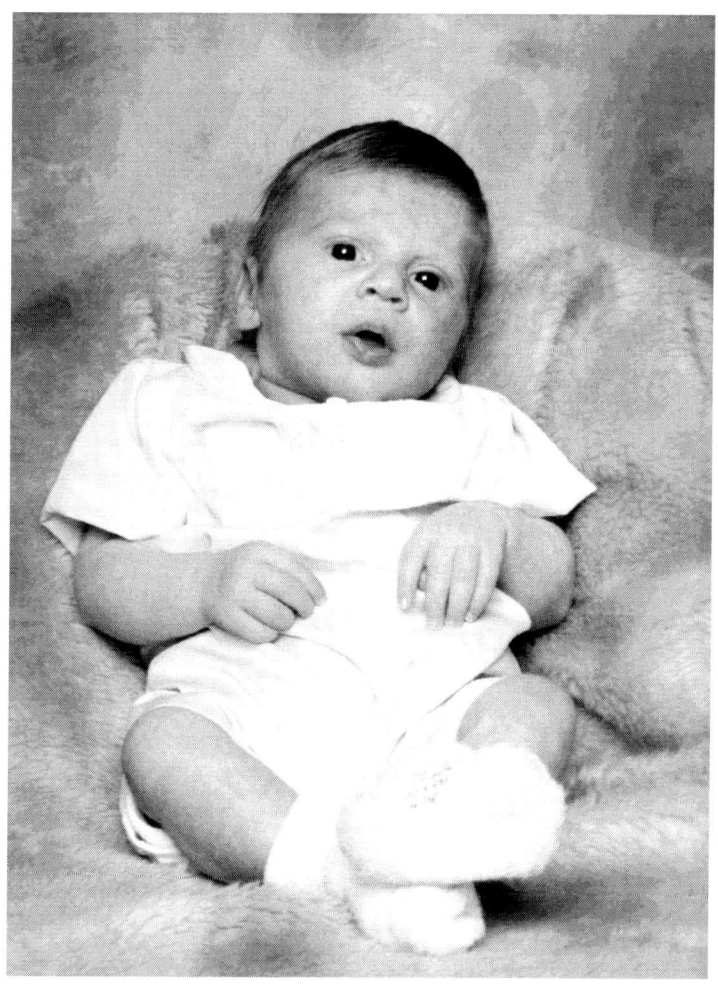

This is me before anyone knew I was ill. Soon after this was taken, I was told that I didn't have long to live. But I fooled them!

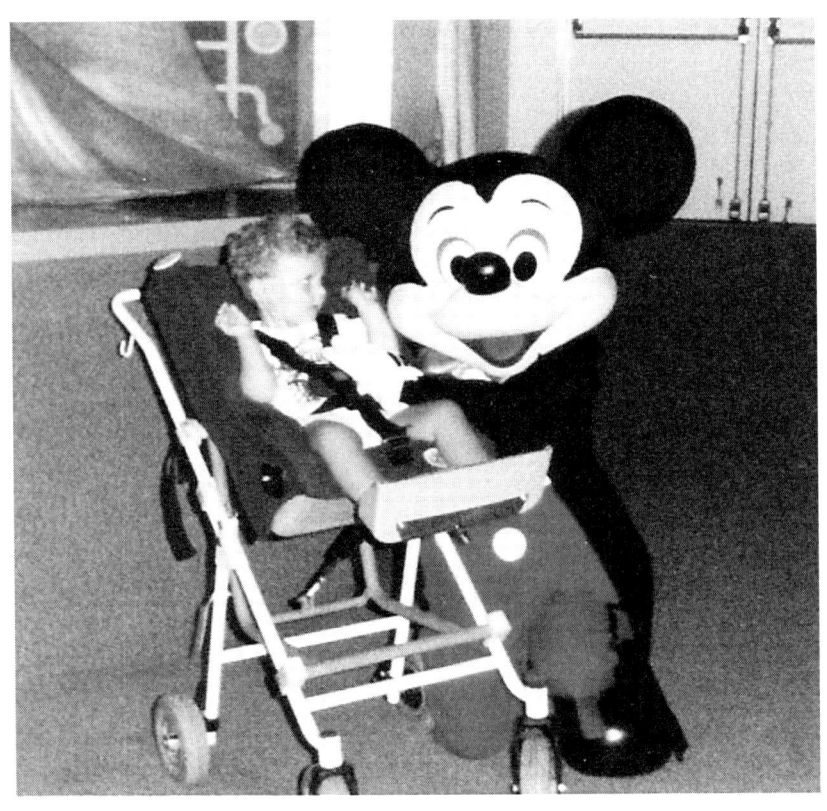

I always wanted to meet Mickey Mouse – and I did on several occasions.

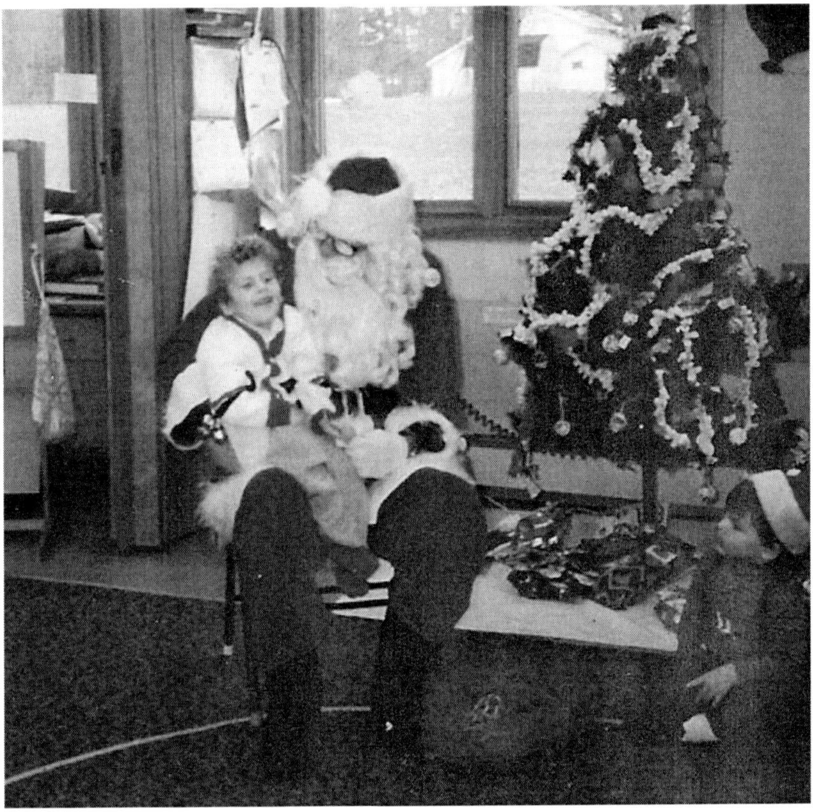

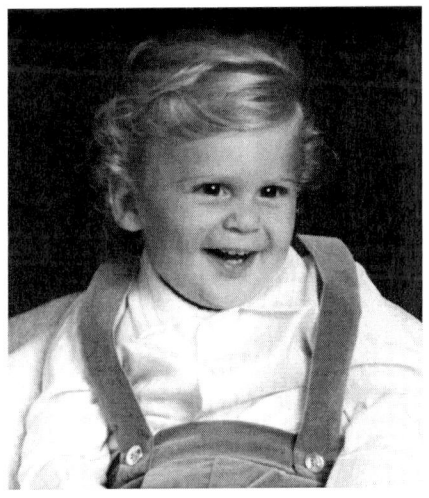

Christmas! What could be better? Here's me with Santa.

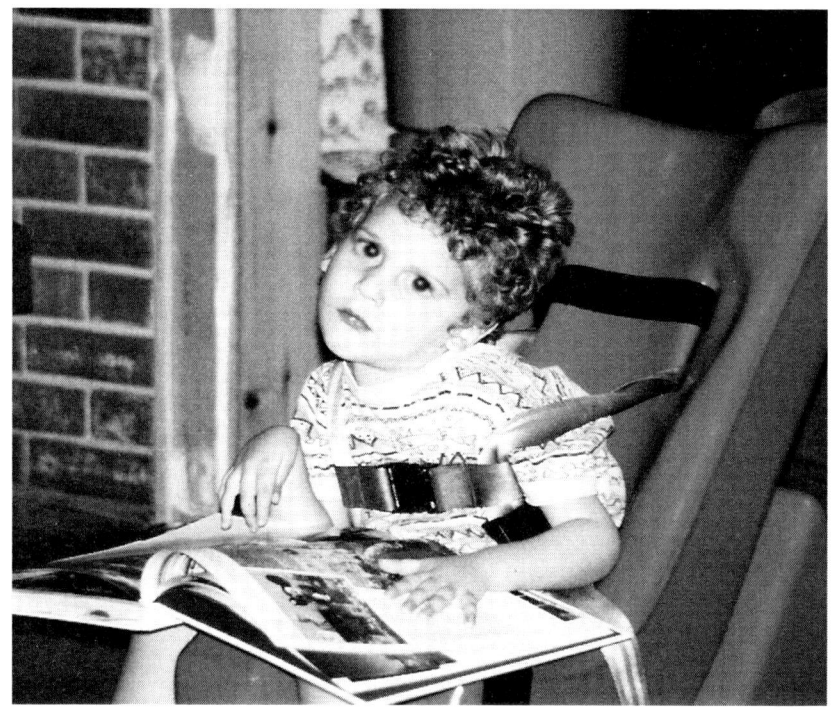

This is a picture of me in my "Tumbleform," a device similar to a baby seat, but designed to give me the support that I needed. I had to be strapped in all the time; and special care was given in order to keep my head upright to prevent me from suffocating. I used my Tumbleform until I was able to sit in a wheelchair.

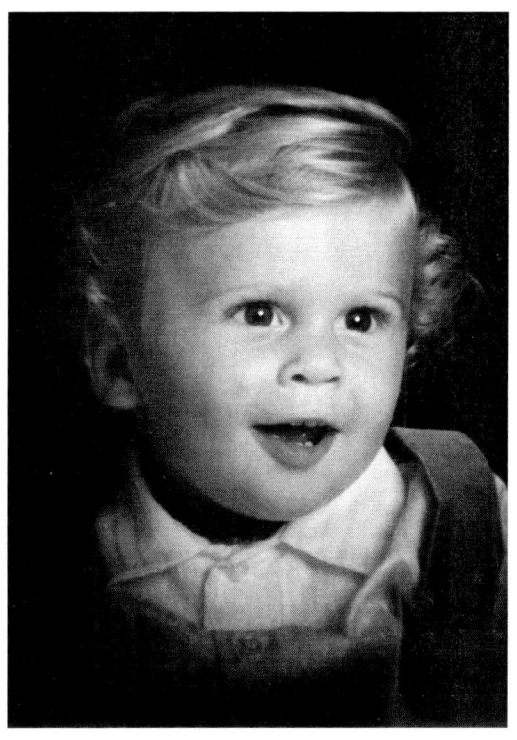

People have told me that I was always smiling. They said I was one of the happiest babies they have ever seen.

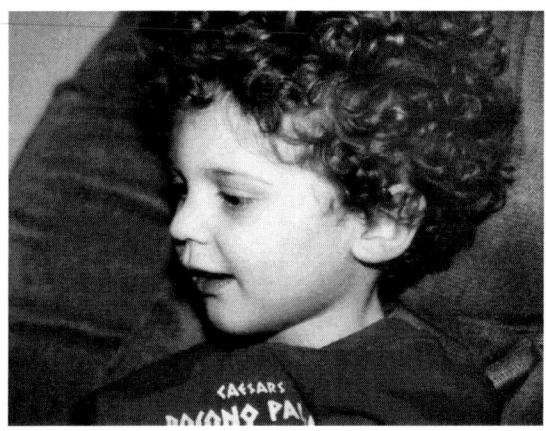

How about that hair!

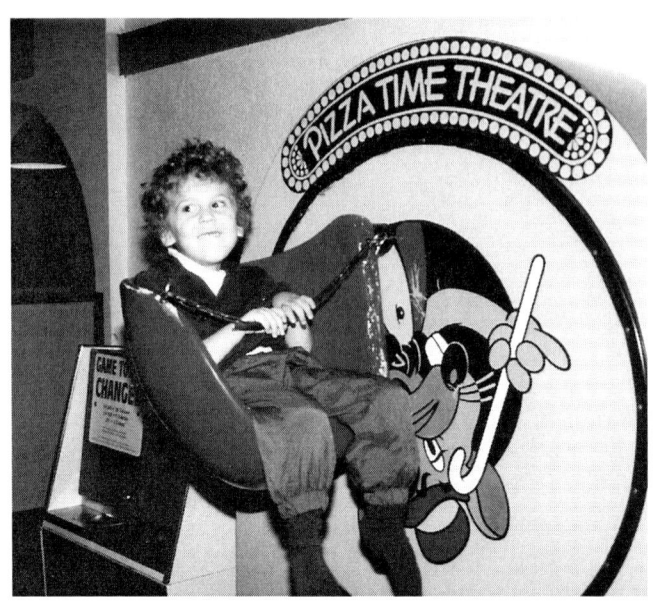

I always like to ride in just about anything, especially if it moved fast!

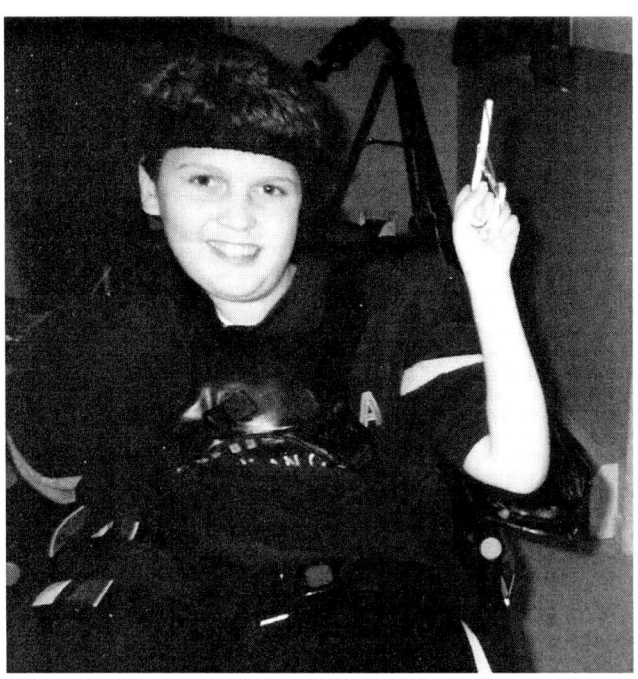

Chapter Ten: Snappy

I always looked forward to the first day of school. New subjects. New faces. New friends. This enthusiasm carried through from September to June – except one year – the worst school year of my life. And it was all because of one woman. It was all because of my teacher.

I call her "Ms. Snappy" because she was short-tempered. She was always yelling at someone. She was always yelling at me. No matter what I did, right or wrong, she was always out to get me, right from the first day of class.

"You," she said. "Yeah, I've been waiting for you." I thought that was a good sign. The teacher already knew me. It wasn't. I thought it meant that my reputation had preceded me. It had. But reputations can be tricky. While I thought my reputation as a good student had filtered its way to Ms. Snappy, it was the reputation for being in a wheelchair that she fixated on. And that caused problems. She seemed to have an issue with the whole idea of inclusion. Maybe she thought that by me being in her class, it would mean more work for her. No matter what it was, she never made me feel welcome there. Not once.

"I want you to sit over there by the window, out of the way. And do not block anyone with that wheelchair of yours. Do you understand me?"

"Yes," I replied. I took my place at the back of the room.

"And your nurse," she added. "She can only sit if we have a spare chair. If not, she stands. Never use a desk meant for a real student."

I got a bad feeling in my stomach, like I was being punished. But for what? Day after day, it was more of the same.

"Stand for the Pledge of Allegiance, class. Except you, Craig. You may stay seated."

It got worse as the year progressed.

"When I call your name, go to the board and finish the next math problem. Everyone gets a turn but Craig. We don't have that much time."

Though I tried my best, I was uncomfortable in her class, and that started affecting my life. My work wasn't as good. My attendance suffered. I had no fun and almost dreaded going to school each day, which wasn't like me at all.

It all came to a head one day. I shall never forget it because it was the single worst day that I had in my entire elementary school life. It was the day that Ms. Snappy tried to break my spirit.

The class had just finished an assignment and handed it in. I did so, too, right on time. I prided myself about doing my work on time – and by myself. A lot of people thought that by having a nurse by my side, they were helping me – or even worse – giving me answers. I can honestly say that that never happened. Not once. And if anyone had offered help, I would have gotten annoyed with them. I wanted the pleasure of doing my work for myself.

A little while after handing the work in, Ms. S. announced that I was being punished.

"Why?" I asked. "What did I do?"

"It's not what you did," she said, "It's what you didn't do."

I had no idea what she meant. It sounded like a riddle.

"You forgot to write your name at the top of the page."

Ms. S. walked over and showed me my work. Sure enough, she was right. I had forgotten to write my name.

"And you know the rules, Craig," she explained. "Tonight for punishment I want you to write your name on a piece of paper 100 times. And I expect this to be handed in first thing tomorrow morning."

What could I say? What could I do? If I complained, if I said that it wasn't fair, then I would be saying that I didn't want to be treated the same as everyone else – and I did.

I felt like screaming and crying and hiding, all at the same time. Of course, I could not do the work. She knew it. I had trouble writing. It took me forever just to write a simple sentence. Lots of people knew that. They accepted it. They didn't make a big deal out of it. Ms. Snappy was the only one who ever had to point it out.

When I got home later that day, I was distraught.

"Why does she hate me, Mom?"

"I don't think she hates you," my mother said.

"I do. She acts like I did something bad to her – like I am bad. I try and I try. Nothing works. She hates me."

"I know you try, Honey. I know you try hard. But you're not bad. Don't ever say that."

"She makes me feel like something is wrong with me; but I

don't feel like there is anything wrong with me. Is there?"

"No, Craig."

"I just don't get it."

"Well, some people are like that. Unfortunately, a lot of people are like that. When your teacher looks at you, she doesn't see you; she sees the chair. And that bothers her. She doesn't see a normal boy. She sees that she has to change the way she thinks and the way she does things in her classroom, and she doesn't like that."

"Because of me?"

"Yes, because of you."

"Because it takes me a long time to write?"

"Yes. That and a million other things. With you there, she has to run her class differently. She has to change her habits and that makes her uncomfortable. That's why she's always angry. She is lazy and likes to stay in her rut and just keeping doing the same thing over and over and over."

"Yeah. The kids don't like that. Sometimes they talk about her behind her back."

"When she sees you, Craig, she sees change. She sees the world changing all around her; and that intimidates her. She's scared, so she fights back by taking it out on you. That's why she always seems angry. That's whys she yells a lot."

"Yeah, for sure."

"In some ways it's just plain old laziness. In some ways it's worse. In some ways it's prejudice."

"You think so?"

"Yes I do. She doesn't want you in her class. It would be easier for her if you weren't there. She would rather not have you around.."

"Dead?"

"No, not dead. Separated from everyone else. Separated from all the so-called normal people."

"But I *am* normal, Mom."

"I know, Craig."

"I *am* normal. It's just *my* normal. Is there anything wrong with that? Am I different? Did God make me different?"

"How can you even ask such a thing?"

"But I can't do everything that the other kids can do. I *am* different. Why did God make me different?"

"Everyone is different," Mom explained. "But being different does not mean that anything is wrong. It means that we are all unique. Yes, you do have a disease, but that's all part of who you are. It's like: Johnny has brown hair or Billy has freckles or Sally has blue eyes. It's part of you. Only in this case we are talking about your muscles. In this case, it's more like: Johnny can run fast, Billy can run slow, and Craig runs in his wheelchair."

I smiled a little.

"It's just one little thing out of all the many things that make up who you are. It's just one little thing out of all the many, many big things of your life. There is nothing wrong with you and you are right to believe that. You will just have to accept the fact that the world is filled with people just like your teacher."

"I can accept it, but I will never like it."

"And you shouldn't."

"Maybe someday things will change. Maybe someday I will make things change."

"I have no doubt about that."

"Mom, did you ever wonder why God made me like this?"

"Yes, a few times," she admitted. "But only God can answer that question. I will say this, though. God does have a plan. He has a plan for everyone and that includes you and me. God made you this way because He loves you and wants you to be part of His plan. The only way we can find out what that reason is, is to live our lives and see where we go. Does that make sense?"

"A little," I said.

"Good," Mom said, smiling. Then she kissed me on the top of the head and said, "Okay, let's take a look at that punishment of yours."

I got help later that night; and the punishment was turned in the very next day, right on time.

Also on that day, my mother marched into the school to have a talk with school officials. She had already had to fight to keep me out of special education classes, as was their plan in the first place. She never wanted that for me, and neither did I. It had worked out fine so far, and she wasn't going to let this mishap derail years of work. Mom was not going to let anyone bully me into anything.

After that, not another word was said. But the pain of that experience still lingers. That was the first time that someone wanted to hurt me on purpose. That was the first time that someone took pleasure in maliciously pointing out that I was incapable of doing something.

Deep inside I felt like saying, "I get it. I get it! I can't do it. You win. I can't do it. Are you happy now?"

The only thing left to do after that was to pick myself up and show people what I *could* do.

Chapter Eleven: The Voice

In the early years of my life, most of my time – when I wasn't sick – was spent with my grandpa. Grandpa was my chauffeur, my teacher, and my buddy. We were inseparable. He took me everyplace I wanted to go and spoiled me whenever he could.

"Who's up for some ice cream?" Grandpa asked, knowing all too well that I never refused ice cream – or a chance to take a trip in the van to get some.

"Me, me, me!"

"Well, then, let's get a move on before it all melts and there's none left for us."

"Can I get chocolate, Grandpa?"

"Yes, you can get chocolate."

"Can I get vanilla, Grandpa?"

"What happened to chocolate?"

"Can I get vanilla after the chocolate?"

"Two cones? Well, maybe if they're small."

"Can I get strawberry, Grandpa?"

"I swear, boy, you're a bottomless pit."

I wound up getting three cones that day, and a bit of a bellyache; but it was worth it.

Grandpa shared his love with everyone. He always had a kind word to say. I can't ever remember hearing him complain about anything, not even about me when I bombarded him with questions or asked him to take me all over the place. He loved his family, his church, and his music.

One afternoon after school when I was in first grade, I was bored out of my mind because all my homework was done and, well, let's just say that I liked to keep busy. I found myself hanging out with my grandpa, although if you really want to be accurate about it, I was probably pestering him to death. Grandpa had his nose buried in the big, red book; and I could tell that he was trying to concentrate, so naturally I had to ask a few questions.

"Hey, Grandpa, whatcha doing?"

At first, he just looked up and smiled. He was used to my interruptions. He continued reading his book. So, that meant that I had to try harder.

"Hey, Grandpa, what's that?"

Grandpa knew that I would not stop unless he gave me a good enough answer, so he put his book down and answered me.

"This is my hymnal, C.V.," he explained.

"Hymnal?" I asked

"Yes. It's from church. It's a big book with hundreds of songs in it. I read it when I have to sing."

"Are you going to sing now?"

That's when Grandpa realized that he had never heard me sing anything much more than a few quiet notes under my breath. Nobody had – and for a good reason. You see, most children with SMA-Type 1, do not have a strong enough voice to sing. Some cannot even speak at all. Everyone in my family was aware of this, and was simply grateful for the fact that I could talk to them. They never considered the thought of testing me out, just to see if I could belt out a few notes. They were always wary of my breathing, my lungs, my throat, and my mouth. They were careful – maybe too careful. So Grandpa got the idea that it just might be time to take a chance.

"Yes and no, C.V.," Grandpa said.

"What do you mean?"

"Well, I will sing a little bit; and then I want you to sing after me."

"Me?"

"Yes, you," he continued. "I think we should just see what you can do. What harm could there be?"

Grandpa opened the hymnal to a random page.

"I will sing a few words and then you try your best to copy me, okay?"

"Okay," I smiled back.

Grandpa cleared his throat, and there, listening to his beautiful tenor voice, began my fascination with music.

"Oh come, oh come Emmanuel," he sang. "Now you try."

I did everything the same way that Grandpa did. I cleared my throat. Then I sang.

"Oh come, oh come, Emmanuel."

Then I waited…and waited…and waited.

Grandpa did not say a word. I assumed that I must have done a bad job.

"Maybe this singing thing is not for me," I thought. I decided to give it another try.

"Oh come, oh come, Emmanuel," I sang, only this time a little louder.

Grandpa started to cry. Then he ran out of the room. I figured that I must have been really bad. I figured that I should stick to watching television. That's when Grandpa showed up again, only now he was tugging my grandmother and nurse into the room.

"Can you sing that one more time?" he asked.

"Oh come, oh come, Emmanuel."

Again the room went silent. I figured that I must be so horrible that Grandpa needed an audience to hear me for themselves, or else no one would believe any of his stories about how bad I was.

Now three people were crying. I was ready to give up. I liked making people laugh, not making them cry.

"Angel!" Grandpa said. "The boy has the voice of an angel!"

"This is not supposed to happen," Grandma added. "This is impossible. The doctors always said…"

"Who cares what the doctors said," Grandpa interrupted. "This is the voice of an angel. We have to share this gift. We have to."

Grandpa took charge. He started teaching me all that he could about music, notes, scales, you name it. He would grab his hymnal and pick his favorites; and then we would sing together, smiling all the while. This was one of the happiest times of my life.

Soon, Grandpa felt that, as he would say, it was time to "take my show on the road." Grandpa wanted me to start singing in public.

During periods of time when I was relatively healthy, I would go all over the place and sing to people. I can remember the first time I sang at church. I was right in front of the choir, sitting in my wheelchair, while my grandma held the microphone to my mouth. I enjoyed this very much except for one thing. Now, instead of just having two or three people crying, I had well over a hundred in tears. Still, they kept telling me that I had a beautiful voice, so I continued to sing.

One time, on Christmas Eve, I was scheduled to sing "Oh, Holy Night" at my church's worship service. My family wasn't sure if I could do it because I was battling through another one of my episodes with pneumonia. But we didn't want to let anyone down, so we decided to give it a try. I guess I figured that God probably didn't want to spoil his Son's birthday by calling me up to Heaven at that point. They wheeled me into church all bundled up and shivering. I stayed just long enough to sing the song. Then they rushed me off to get medical attention, as they could see I was getting worse – and fast. But once again, this brush with death was only a close call. Once again I got better.

Grandpa thought it was important that I study music so that I could get better at it. My family decided to enroll me at the William Michael Center for the Arts, where I began keyboard and voice lessons. This involved lots and lots of practice, which I enjoyed because I liked to keep busy. I had a small, electric keyboard that was placed across my lap. It was difficult for me to move my fingers to hit the right notes, but I kept practicing anyway.

I remember only one recital, where I played the Star Wars theme song by myself, and everyone said nice things about me. But I was not real enthused or passionate about playing the keyboard, so I only took the lessons for a little over a year. But I was a good singer, and enjoyed that very much, so my voice lessons continued.

There are several other important memories that I have when I look back to my musical life. When I was only nine years old, I was asked to sing the National Anthem at P & C Stadium to open a baseball game for the Syracuse Sky Chiefs, our local minor league team. All of my friends and family drove down to the stadium to watch me.

I was wheeled into a special entrance to the stadium and led onto the field, just like a V.I.P. I made my way behind home plate, where someone held a microphone for me. I looked around at the hundreds and hundreds of people, drew as big a breath as I could, and belted out my best rendition of "The Star Spangled Banner." Afterwards, the crowd applauded and there were cheers – and even some of the players came up to me to compliment me and say hello.

I became the youngest person ever to sing the National Anthem at a Chiefs' game. It was a blast!

My voice kept getting stronger and stronger as the singing lessons continued. I was taught breathing techniques that allowed me to hold more breath in my lungs so I could hold the notes longer. I practiced these techniques over and over again because I wanted to sing as well as Grandpa, who sat with me for hours, carefully helping me with my breathing and my scales. Sometimes we would sing harmony. That was the best!

This was where my love of music began, with Grandpa by my side, just the two of us in my room. In my mind it was as simple as that – love of music. My love of music made me want to practice more and more. Years later, my doctor told me that all my breathing exercises strengthened my lungs and kept me off ventilators, helped me battle pneumonia and stave off infections. My love of music helped save my life.

Chapter Twelve: Sharing Gifts

I wanted to make sure that I continued studying music and sharing my singing well after the summer had ended. To me, my singing was not a causal thing – it was important. When school started up again, I asked to be allowed to join the chorus – and they said yes! Now I was singing regularly in front of large crowds. Nothing felt better than that – except for what I was able to do with my singing for my mother.

Right before I started the sixth grade, my mom remarried, and I received a wonderful stepdad, along with a great new family. I also sang during their wedding. Then, at the reception, while my grandparents were giving Mom and Dad their gift, I surprised them with another song. My sister Cralynne, who was eight at the time, held the microphone for me while I sang "The Rainbow Connection."

Mom was speechless and in tears. And I got the biggest hugs and kisses from everyone. It was a magic moment in our lives. I have always felt happy to have been able to give something to her, after all that she has done for me. To this day, Mom still says that the video of me singing that song is her favorite video of all time.

By the time sixth grade rolled around, I was beginning to think that life was getting too easy, if you can imagine that. Sixth grade was my time to shine. After all, sixth graders are the big shots. We rule the school. The little kids look up to you. Besides, everyone – and I do mean everyone – knew me. I was very hard to miss.

I had lots of friends. Why, I even had people pretending to be my friends, just so they could hang out with me. They usually fell into a few easy-to-spot categories. First, there were my true friends. These were the kids who ate with me in the cafeteria, came to my house, played games, shared stories, and did all the things – good and bad – that friends normally do.

Next, we had what I call my "protectors." These were the kids who wanted to take care of me. They were concerned about my safety. They kept crowds at an arm's length; and always made sure my needs were met. They were especially good at shooing away the dumb little kids who always wanted to touch my chair, just to see what it felt like out of curiosity.

There was also a large group of kids who wanted to get close to me for other reasons. One of these was because they thought that a wheelchair was cool. I guess that when they saw me darting around the gym in my chair, it seemed like a 3-D video game come to life. To them, being close to someone cool would make them cool by osmosis. To be honest, they didn't serve much purpose to me. I tolerated them just to be polite.

The last group of kids were the ones who drifted to me out of curiosity. Mostly comprised of the very young, these kids bombarded me with question after question in a non-stop interview about my daily life.

"How does it feel to be in a wheelchair?"

"How fast can you go in that thing?"

"What happens if it gets wet? Do you get a shock?"

"Can I go for a ride?"

"Do you need a license to drive that?"

You get the idea.

There was another group of kids who liked to hang out by my side, following me wherever I went. That group was girls.

Girls were intrigued by my situation. Girls flocked to me like I was giving away free candy or something. I don't know if they loved the chair, if they felt extra-protective of me, or if they just wanted to see if I could feel it when they touched me (which I could,) but that didn't matter. I could never have too many girls around.

Despite my comfort with elementary school (and apparent fame), I entered the sixth grade with a little trepidation. That's because I had heard that my soon-to-be teacher was mean. I was assigned to the dreaded Mr. D.

The information from the school grapevine said that Mr. D. didn't tolerate any kind of fooling around in class, he was constantly yelling, and that no one had any fun.

"Don't mess with Mr. D.," was the prevailing feeling at school. "You'll be sorry if you do."

I thought back to Ms. Snappy and how I felt back then. I didn't want a repeat performance of that disaster of a school year. So, for the first time in my life, I was a little nervous.

Boy, was I dead wrong. Sixth grade was the single best year of elementary school.

I can still remember that first day, as I entered the room with a lump in my throat. Mr. D. greeted me at the door and told me to follow him to my seat.

"I don't know how they did it in your other classes, Craig," he explained, "but this is how we are going to do it in my class."

"Oh no," I thought. *"It's Ms. Snappy, all over again."*

"First of all," he explained, "I don't want you sitting in the back of the room – ever. I want you right in the middle of things with everyone else. I want you to try your best to do what all of my students do: assignments, class work, writing at the board…everything."

That didn't sound too bad to me. In fact, it was exactly what I wanted to do and how I wanted to be treated. I began to think that all the gossip might be wrong. Then, Mr. D. introduced himself to the class and laid down a few rules in his firm, but friendly voice.

"Some people say that I am strict," he said. "I know all the rumors. I have heard all the stories."

I looked around to see if anyone else was scared. I saw a lot of nervous faces.

"There is a big difference between being strict and being fair. I think you will find that I am very, very fair."

Mr. D. went on to explain about respect, and how people should treat everyone else. His words were welcome ones to my ears. His attitude was the same as mine. I immediately felt like this was going to be a great year. And I was right.

Later on that school year, Mr. D. had one of his many talks

with me. He explained his teaching philosophy. He told me that he never wanted a single student to feel invisible. He said that he was well aware of how that could happen to someone in my situation, and how the easy thing to do would be to try to push us aside or ignore us. He said that he always tried to picture what it would be like for his own child to be in a wheelchair. He wanted for me the same things that he wanted for a child of his own. He wanted me to feel like I belonged, like I was supposed to be here.

Mr. D. was more than a teacher to me. What I learned from him went far beyond the classroom. Mr. D. taught me about life. Sure, I learned a lot about developing good study habits and a solid work ethic; but I also learned just as much about people and how we should treat one another.

For instance, I can remember one time when I was talking to Mr. D. The conversation was nothing special, just one of our usual chats that somehow always had a hidden lesson for me in there somewhere. During the conversation, I thanked him for all that he had taught me. And that's when he said something that has stuck with me to this day.

"Craig," he said, "I have learned just as much from you as you have learned from me."

That's my idea of perfection.

Even though things were going my way at school, that doesn't mean that my life was ever easy. Struggle was always involved. No matter what anyone did, no matter how careful everyone was, I was always getting ill. It simply could not be prevented.

I always got pneumonia – always. This happened to me several times each year, and I had to be pulled out of school until I recovered. And although I was used to this alternating pattern of illness and health, I dreaded it because it hurt so much. To get me to breathe, the nurses actually had to pound on my chest over and over again. This would loosen the phlegm, which hopefully I would then cough up. These episodes left me bruised and sore; and it left the nurses tired. I would sometimes lie in bed for hours, trying to ignore the pain in my body and the sadness in my heart from being away from my friends at school. I simply could not wait to return, even if it meant tons and tons of homework, just to catch up with the rest of the class – and I always did.

By the time summer arrived, my life was again in a good place. Even though I hated to leave Mr. D. and elementary school, I was excited about the new challenges that junior high school would bring. Elementary school had given me the opportunity to feel comfortable and to branch out and try many things. I always thought that each step along the way would be the same. I was naive. Even though I was beginning to become worldly, I had no sense of what was in store along the way. But others did.

I can remember a serious talk I had with Mr. D., right after our trip to visit the junior high school. The class had been taken there for an orientation guide around the school, just to familiarize us with what we would be encountering the upcoming year. Mr. D. admitted to me that he was scared for me the whole time.

"Craig," he said with sadness in his eyes, "I have always told it to you straight and I am not going to stop now."

His words sounded serious.

"I have always wanted you to be a part of everything in my class. This is true. But the world is not always like my class. Sometimes it can be rough. People can be mean. People can be abusive."

I had no idea what he meant, but I listened to every single word.

"Please be careful. Be very, very careful next year. Junior high is a different world."

And he was oh, so right.

Chapter Thirteen: The Mob

The summer prior to entering junior high school was warm and inviting; just like the late afternoon breeze that blew across Lake Neahtawanta, where I often sat with my grandfather. We'd watch the geese ripple the orange and red water as the sun slowly sank, saying good night to Fulton. I could feel my life changing as I straddled the days between boyhood and manhood. I grew comfortable and confident in my wheelchair, and found it much easier to become independent – or as independent as I could ever be with the 24-hour care I always needed. I looked forward to the next school year with eagerness and nervous anticipation. New routines – changing classes instead of staying put in one classroom – new people, new challenges. I knew that I could handle them. After all, I was no longer a kid. I was an elementary school graduate.

Also during that summer, I spent a lot of time at my family's church. I guess you could say that we have always been a religious family, but that isn't really why I went to church so often. If I didn't like going – if it didn't feel right to me – I would have resisted in my own stubborn way. But the fact of the matter is that it *did* feel right to me. I enjoyed most everything about it: the people, the pastor, the fun and, especially, the music.

Right about mid-summer, my church held something called "Vacation Bible School." This was sort of like a summer camp that was held over an entire week each evening. The grownups from the church went all out to schedule games, activities, arts and crafts, and lots of snacks and music for the young people of the community. A large crowd usually showed up; and I just loved all the fun and excitement. And to be perfectly honest, I also loved racing the other kids around the church. Lots of times they had to calm me down because I would almost get too excited, as if that's possible.

I had been to many Vacation Bible Schools since I was able to get around, but this year's was quite different. In the others, I was content to laugh and sing and gobble up the sugary-sweet snacks. But not in this V.B.S. In this V.B.S. I had a hard time concentrating on the activities. My mind was someplace else. And it was all because she was there.

Her name was Becca. Now before you jump to conclusions, let me set the record straight. This wasn't a case of Becca being the first girl I had ever noticed. Far from it. I was always surrounded by girls. In fact, they loved to touch me. I can distinctly remember a lot of girls (and women) saying something about my hands having "the softest skin that they have ever felt." Even today, members of the female gender still come up to me and ask to feel my hands. So whether it was my hands, the chair, or the need to "mother" me, as far as females were concerned, I was magnetic.

I would also like to point out that my feelings for Becca weren't "puppy love" or whatever cliché you'd like to apply. This was completely different. Becca was unlike any girl I had ever seen before. She had beautiful, blonde hair, almost to her shoulders, with a gentle curl in it right below her chin. It was if the sun itself directed you to follow its beams down her head and then up again until you got a glimpse of her striking eyes and enchanting smile. And, oh, what a smile – so bright and warm that it would make the sun jealous.

The first few days of Vacation Bible School, I just stared at her. It was all that I could do. Still I knew that Becca was no ordinary girl and that this was the very first time that I had ever felt serious about anyone. So, I had to do something or else I would have felt like a fool. It was hard to imagine, me, a man of the world, a sixth-grade graduate, a regular chatterbox, being unable to figure out how to approach a girl, or what words to say when I got the nerve to finally do so, but that's exactly how it was. I was frozen. Frozen by this vision with the amazing smile.

I finally got the courage to tell someone how I felt about Becca. I had to, because I needed help. I eventually had a friend approach her to let her know I was interested. I wish I could say that this is a "happily ever after" story. But it isn't. As I had suspected, Becca wasn't interested in me. I wasn't really sure why; but at that point, I did not want to find out. It hurt enough being rejected from afar. I saw no need to inflict any more pain upon myself. So I gave up on Becca, and that was that…for the time being.

Summer finally ended and the chill of autumn arrived. Autumn is a gorgeous time of year in Central New York. The trees seem to burst to life with color, singing their sweetest melody just before they die. I have always thought that this was the best way to live. You get better all the time until the day comes when you are gone. That's the way to do it. Autumn also sees the nights starting to get colder, which has always been a reminder to me that harsh "Old Man Winter" is right around the bend, and that some adult is soon going to force me to wear a jacket. But I didn't pay much attention to all of that. I was too excited about moving up to junior high school.

The first thing I remember about my first day of junior high school is that my transportation took a giant leap forward. I have always been keenly interested in movement, in going places, in getting around (and usually as fast as possible.) So when I graduated from elementary school to junior high school, I not only advanced in grade, I advanced in mobility. Instead of having to ride on a bus (uncool), I now was being transported to school in a van that had been adapted to carry me in my chair (definitely much cooler.)

My grandpa was my driver and he did a great job of getting me to school right on time. He got to pull the van right up close to the building, rush around back, and help me get out by operating the mechanical lift that I used to get up and down. The whole process sometimes attracted a crowd, but I didn't mind. I felt more like a famous person getting out of a limousine than anything else. I liked the attention, especially if it meant more girls would become fans.

I would not describe the first few weeks of junior high school as being smooth. In fact, they were very unsettling and nerve-wracking. They had told us that junior high school was supposed to prepare us for high school. Well, if that meant chaos, confusion, and confrontation, then I would not be so eager to move ahead at all.

When the new seventh graders arrived at school, we were all herded into the cafeteria, where the orientation and introduction process began. There we were divided into three "teams," the Red Team, the White Team, and the Green Team (our three school colors.) The kids that were on your team were the kids that you would see all the time. They would be in your classes, your lunch period, everything. If your best friend had been put on a different team from you, well, you were out of luck. And if your worst enemy had been put on the same team as you, well, then you were even more out of luck.

At first, I started feeling stressed because we now had to change classes. Instead of sitting comfortably in one classroom and letting the teacher worry about getting everyone to where they needed to be, we had to do this on our own – and in only four minutes time between classes. The result was exactly as you might expect: hundreds of kids scrambling to get their books and trying to find a path through a mass of humanity, all frantically jostling and elbowing and shoving. And all of this was taking place while the teachers stood in the hallways and told us not to run, but also not to be late for class.

This was junior high: high energy, strange faces, unfriendly stares, stress. After three weeks, I really needed something to help me start feeling better. And it happened. Just like it had appeared before, music once again entered my life. But this time, its role was even bigger.

I was thrilled to find out that I had been selected to join the junior high school chorus. I loved to sing. I needed to sing. I could not imagine life without music. The chorus was where I belonged.

I'm not sure if you would say that it's difficult to be selected to be in chorus, but not everyone makes it. You have to go through somewhat of an audition process. In the spring of your 6th grade year, the Chorus Director, Mrs. C., would visit all of the elementary schools in Fulton and listen to all of the students sing. Out of all those kids, she would then choose enough of them to fill the chorus, which usually had between 80 and 90 students. I figured that I had a good shot. And I was right.

As soon as I entered the chorus room, I knew I was home. It was just filled wall-to-wall with everything to do with music. There was a huge piano in the center and music stands all over the place. Toward the back wall there were risers, where the students would stand to sing. It even had enough space for me to sit comfortably in my chair, while my nurse sat behind me and enjoyed the show.

In some ways, the chorus room was like an oasis. It felt different in there than in some of the other places in junior high school. The kids acted better toward one another. It didn't seem competitive or mean-spirited, just the opposite. Everyone went out of their way to help each other out. A lot of that is due to the environment that Mrs. C. worked so hard to create. She had a love for music and was very serious about it, just like me. Some people said she was strict. I guess that's true, if setting down some rules and sticking to them so that you can accomplish something means that you are strict. But I didn't see it that way. I saw it as stress-free fun without any worry. I saw it as freedom.

When I sang, my mind became totally focused on the music. It drew me in and held me with a hug almost as warm and comforting as my mother's. My eye rarely wandered. I took in the notes. I felt them reverberate inside me. I loved the whole experience. It used my entire body as nothing else did.

Although I had already realized that I could belt out a tune, it never quite had the impact how powerful a gift this was until my time in the 7th Grade Chorus. Mrs. C. had decided, and everyone else agreed, that I should be a featured soloist during our concerts. I was told that, for many reasons, it was rare to be selected to do this. First of all, most kids did not want the attention that it would draw to be out there on your own, alone, singing an entire song all by yourself. That did not bother me at all. In fact, I loved it. I was an old pro at it; and I enjoyed every minute.

During our first concert, I got to sing "Danny Boy" to a packed room. That song had always appealed to me; and I especially enjoyed hitting the high notes. They sent chills down the listener's spine. My music was laid out in front of me, spread over two music stands. I took a deep breath and waited for my cue from Mrs. C. at the piano. And then I sang.

I didn't look at the audience much, as I was busy focusing on my music. But when the song was done and I looked up, all I could see was everyone standing up with a lot of people wiping their eyes. And they were cheering…and cheering. It was almost embarrassing. But I did manage a smile simply because it felt so amazingly wonderful. There is no other way to describe it. I was in love with my music. I was in love with sharing it with everyone.

I continued to have the opportunity to share my love of music with people from all over. I was chosen to be in the Select Chorus and the All-County Chorus. And I got to sing at a lot of places all over Central New York. It was a lot of fun, but not as much as just being in the chorus room with everyone laughing and singing and hanging on Mrs. C.'s every word.

One day while at chorus, for some strange reason, a little voice inside me told me to look around. I did. I always listened to that voice because you might miss something if you didn't. I am so glad that I did on that day, because right there – just across the room from me – was Becca. This came as a welcome surprise to me. I was happy that I would be able to see her all the time; but I still remembered her words. How can you forget when someone tells you they are "not interested?" You can't. So I just sat there and admired her from afar, never giving up the last glimmer of hope that someday she might change her mind.

Soon, things started to settle down – well as much as anything can ever settle down in junior high school. I was becoming accustomed to the routine and the hustle-bustle. I was becoming accustomed to the frenzied pace, the jostling and bumping, the insults and foul language, and to seeing my nurses trying to keep up with it all. It wasn't easy for them either.

A month into the school year an announcement came over the loudspeaker that the junior high was having its first dance. I had never been to a dance before. I wasn't sure if I should go or not. I asked my grandpa what he thought, and of course he said that

105

whatever I wanted to do was fine. Still, I was undecided. I didn't want to feel like an outsider or an outcast. So I did the best thing I could do. I spoke to my mom about the idea.

"Grandpa tells me that you have something you want to ask me," Mom said one evening right after dinner.

"Yeah, well, I guess I do," I managed to mutter.

"Craig, is something wrong?" she asked. "I have never known you to be at a loss for words."

"I'm not. Not really," I said. "I have a good idea about what I want to do. But I'm just not sure. I guess I feel a little nervous about what might happen."

"Since when did you ever feel nervous? I have never known you to be nervous – not even when you were sick. Oh sure, you got butterflies now and then, but nervous? Nope. Not you. This must be serious."

"Yeah, it's kind of serious," I admitted.

"So, tell me about it."

I had made up my mind long ago to tell Mom about the dance, but not to tell her everything. We shared a lot of things, but I wasn't sure if she was ready to hear that I had feelings for a girl.

"They're having a dance at school…"

No sooner than the word "dance" came out of my mouth, my mom smiled. She was even smarter than I had ever given her credit for.

"And I just don't know if I should go. I mean, I might want to go, but what would I wear?. What would I do, what –"

"Honey," she asked, "forget about all that. There is only one question that matters. Do you want to go? Look into your heart and find the answer. Your heart always tells you what to do. Does it tell you that you want to go?"

Of course it did. I was absolutely aching to go to a dance. I couldn't stop thinking that Becca might be there.

"Yes, Mom, I want to go," I admitted.

"Then that's that. You're going."

"But what about…"

"Forget about everything else. We will make it work. Take your mind off of all of that. We will make it work."

And it did work.

Mom made sure that I had nice clothes to wear. She did a great job, too, picking out clothes that were right in the middle between the overly-formal tuxedo (which did cross my mind) and the dorkiness of gym clothes (which definitely did not.) My outfit was casual and cool, but better than the regular clothes that I wore to school. Just perfect.

I felt more confident now that I had the support of my family and friends. But that confidence waned as soon as I entered the dance. It was as if I had been dropped off on Mars. The gym had been decorated. Music was playing. They even had snacks there. But those were all minor details in comparison to what I was worrying about. I was worrying about what to do and how to fit in.

There were a few kids dancing, but for the most part, people just hung out in groups; the boys on one side and the girls on the other. A few brave boys were on the dance floor, moving about with some girls. I say "moving about" because I wouldn't exactly call what they were doing dancing. A few girls were dancing with each other. I tried not to dwell on that because there was no way that I could dance. I wasn't even sure if I should go onto the dance floor. I did not want the attention if I was going to look like a fool. I felt awkward. I did not know what to do, so I just drove around wishing that I could dance, feeling sorry for myself.

About halfway through the dance, still aimlessly wandering about, feeling like a third shoe, one of Becca's friends approached me.

Oh, no, I thought, *I bet Becca saw me staring at her. I bet she thinks I'm a stalker. I bet she wants to tell me to bug off.*

She handed me a little white piece of paper. It had a number on it.

"She wants you to call her," she said and then quickly walked away.

I was stunned. I was speechless. After all this time. After all this wasted worry. She came to me.

She wants me to call her. She wants me to call her.

Chapter Fourteen: Becca

I spent the next few hours in a daze, trying to figure out how not to blow it. What would I say? How would I break the ice? What could we talk about? And how could I do all this with my nurse holding the phone to my ear? It's hard to feel cool when all those thoughts are running through your head.

It seemed like it took forever; but I finally worked up the guts to give Becca a call. And much to my surprise, she was easy to talk to...and talk to...and talk to. We talked about school and what teachers we liked and didn't like. We talked about food. We talked about music. We talked until my nurse said her phone-holding arm was getting a muscle cramp. That was my signal that it was time to hang up.

Becca and I started hanging out together at school every possible second that we could. When we were in class together, we could hardly stop staring at one another. When we weren't, she would run to where I was just to be able to spend a few minutes together between classes. In chorus, the other kids' voices all seemed mute to me. All I could hear was Becca's. And every time she smiled at me, it was like winning the lottery on my birthday.

If you have been paying attention up to now, you can probably anticipate what I am going to say next. That's right. Becca became my girlfriend.

Though the world of junior high school – something that up until then had not thrilled me – was known to have its fair share of bullies and otherwise unpleasant people, I was finally beginning to learn the ropes and become comfortable with my place amongst the chaos. When I needed to escape, I had the peaceful solace of my music and of Becca. The world began looking good again: I had a girlfriend.

Our telephone chats grew longer and more frequent. Becca was so easy to talk to and so much fun that time stood still while we were connected electronically. Soon our relationship grew, as well as the muscles of the poor souls who had to hold the receiver to my ear. My entourage began looking like a team of weightlifters.

Not being able to get enough of one another, Becca and I decided to take our relationship to the next level – well the next level as far as 7th graders go. We decided that we needed to go out on a date.

Most of what we did could probably be labeled as "hanging out," but it didn't feel like that to us. It felt like so much more. To us, our time together was like a spaceship to the stars: magical, romantic, and miles away from everyone else. We were comfortable together and connected. It was bliss.

At first, we spent a lot of time at my place because of all the conveniences that were there and since it was easy for me get around. Sometimes we would watch television or listen to music. Other times we felt like doing a little bit more. Luckily, everyone understood, and they allowed me to have a little privacy. Instead of being in the room with me, my nurses would leave, but be close enough to come running in case I needed assistance.

It was at times like that when I first noticed that a wheelchair can be a nuisance. It's pretty hard to get close to a girl with 400 pounds of metal wrapped around you. As far as my wheelchair was concerned, if I wanted to snuggle, it was a bruise factory – you can't wrap your arms around a wheelchair. I was alone in that chair, and no one could get close. That was unacceptable. But here I was also lucky to be surrounded by such understanding people. When Becca and I wanted to be alone together and to be close, my nurse would physically place me onto a big chair or sofa right next to her and I would instantly melt into her body, my head so comfortably resting upon her shoulder. I felt like I could spend eternity in that spot.

Becca's family also was very understanding and did everything they could to accommodate our needs. Her father actually took the time out to build a wheelchair ramp at their house just so I could come visit them. This was the first time that I had ever been to a girl's house and it felt great. I felt like an adult.

Time passed and things between us were as wonderful as ever, but soon a few thoughts started becoming frequent visitors to my mind. I began to go through a growth spurt, and this left my body weaker than ever. I had always been unable to control my head and sometimes it would fall forward and cut off my breathing. The nurses always kept a close eye for this, because when it happened I was unable to call for help. If they ever left me for any length of time – a minute or two – they could come back and find me dead. And now my head was getting bigger and growing heavier, so the risk was increasing.

I was also frustrated, not by how it felt, but by what it did to my life. I wanted to spend more time out of my chair, but that was starting to become dangerous. I couldn't support myself at all. It was hard to prop me up. It prevented me from doing things. And one of those things was getting close to Becca.

I can remember day after day thinking about what could happen, what might happen, what I wanted to happen. But I was helpless to initiate anything. I had to sit there and wait and dream and hope. For a boy my age, this was not an easy task.

But, it did happen.

It was a quiet afternoon and we were alone in my room. We didn't have much to say to each other that day. Our eyes did all the talking. Becca looked at me. I looked back. Looking at Becca was as enjoyable as my music. Both made me feel totally alive.

Becca didn't look the same that day. Something was different. I was in my chair and she was walking around the room casually, almost as if her mind was someplace else, as she fiddled through CDs. She looked down at the floor and then up at me, over and over. And then she stopped.

Her gaze became more intent. She took a step toward me. Then another. Our eyes never parted as she slowly drew near to me, her face just inches from mine. And then it happened. We shared our first kiss.

I am told that everyone remembers their first kiss. I certainly do. I felt like Neil Armstrong stepping onto the moon or Columbus discovering America. I had set foot in a new world. I don't know if everyone's first kiss is good or not. Mine was, for sure. But the best part of it was that it was shared with someone as special as Becca.

Becca and I were together for eight long and wonderful months, a lifetime at that age. Since then we have both moved on, but have been friendly toward one another. We still occasionally talk, catch up on things, and remember all the good times we shared together. I will never forget my wonderful Becca, my first kiss – my first love.

Chapter Fifteen: Rebellion

After our breakup, I was unsettled and confused. I did not understand how something so wonderful could become so bad this quickly. I could not think straight. I never saw it coming. I felt as if I had been blindsided. I began to wonder if there were signs that I should have seen, something that would have signaled we were going in the wrong direction. I missed Becca; I missed her like nothing I have ever missed before.

This was the first time I had ever experienced such a loss. This was the first time that I had my heart broken. And because I did not understand how I was supposed to deal with these feelings, I began to do some pretty irrational things. I questioned everything. I became moody and started acting out. My grades started falling and I didn't care one bit. I just was not interested or motivated to do anything.

I began testing the limits to see what I could get away with. I had noticed long ago that some people would see the wheelchair and look the other way, which is something that I hated. They only saw the chair, as if it was my identity. They never bothered to see me. Others did, but felt only pity for me, which also bothered me. They didn't see me as a normal person. They let me get away with things that they would never allow a so-called normal person to do. So I figured it was time to take advantage of that. I felt that if that's the way they wanted to treat me, then it was their problem and they'd have to figure out a way to deal with it.

Oh, I was never disruptive or evil in that sense, especially in class. But once in a while I might bump into something with my chair – accidentally on purpose – or drop something, just to see what the reaction would be. And of course, there was none. It seemed like no one had the guts to punish me. That just made me feel worse. That just made me act out more.

One day I did the unthinkable. I acted out in Mrs. C.'s class. I entered the chorus room with a huge wad of chewing gum in my mouth, two or three pieces, if I remember correctly. Then, I proceeded to chew it as blatantly as possible, loudly and with my mouth wide open, just to make sure she would not be able to miss me. Mrs. C. had strict rules about chewing gum, so I wanted to see if she would give me the same punishment as the other kids.

It didn't take long to find out. Mrs. C. immediately came over, confiscated my gum, and marked me down for chewing gum in class. Then, she scolded me. Since this was my first offense, there was no big penalty. That came after you did three things wrong, which was definitely not in my plans…yet.

I know it sounds weird, but I was very happy to get punished. Being punished helped me to start feeling the same as everyone else again, and that was just what I needed. So I started settling down in class as far as the teachers were concerned. But if you were a student, look out!

I have to admit that I did some pretty aggressive stuff for a while. I guess it was because my chair made me feel invincible. If I got in someone's face, well, what were they going to do about it? Hit me? I doubt it. And even if they did – and even if I got hurt – I always had others around me to back me up, or my nurse to pick up the pieces. For a while, I was Superman, though I behaved more like Darth Vader.

Once, while in class, this jerk was on my case. This guy had had it in for me for quite a while, something that was not uncommon in the day-to-day junior high school life. He was always making some wise crack about me, saying just enough to make my blood boil deep inside. One day he went way too far.

"Hey, Wheel-boy, did you do the assignment?"

"Yeah, I got it done."

"So who helped you this time, your nurse or your mommy?"

"I did it myself."

"Yeah, right. You did it yourself."

"I did."

"Yeah, sure, and next you'll be telling me that you're going out for the track team."

That was below the belt, so I ignored it.

"You know as well as I do that you get away with murder around here."

"I do not!"

"Always getting special treatment. Everybody does everything for you. And for what? Just because you are physically handicapped. You're pathetic."

I could take being teased. I could take being kidded or even being called stupid or ugly. But nobody gets away with calling me handicapped. Luckily – for him – all I needed to do was to cut him down to size.

"I'd rather have my physical handicap than your mental handicap."

He looked at me, stunned. He wasn't sure what to do. Charge me? Hit me? Try to push me over? I didn't care. Fortunately for him, the teacher entered the room and that put an end to it.

He was lucky. Others weren't. Just after that fight almost happened, I got even closer to another physical confrontation. This one had been building up for quite some time, only now my pent up frustration from losing Becca caused me to snap and attack.

This time my foe was the school bully (one of several, and I despised them all.) He was merciless in his attacks and relentless in his persistence. And he always sought out the weakest and most vulnerable in school. He beat people up, teased, stole their money, everything. He ran the complete gamut of offenses in the bully "how-to" handbook. And, since I must have appeared weak or needy to him, he didn't like me one bit. I must say that the feeling was mutual.

I hated the way that he treated me, and I hated the way that he treated others. And for quite some time I had been having the urge to put him in his place. The biggest problem was that he was clever. He was sneaky. He would walk past you in the hallway and mutter some insult under his breath, just loud enough for you to hear, yet inaudible to any nearby teacher. And he loved to do this as close to a teacher as possible, because if you went after him to retaliate, it would appear as if you had started the whole thing. When no one was around, it was a different story. Then he would just pound you with his fists.

116

He had been on my case for weeks, calling me names, giving me dirty looks. Little did he realize how much rage I had been storing. Then, one day, he made the fatal mistake of using the "H" word. He knew that I didn't like to be called handicapped, even if it was the correct thing to say. That didn't matter. I just didn't like that word. So he used it, and used it a lot.

Then, I completely snapped. It happened in the hallway when no teachers were around. He walked past me with that irritating walk, called me what I hated to be called, turned around and confronted me with a stare-down. And I gave it back to him. We stared at each other for a while; and then he smiled.

And then I charged.

I floored the throttle of my wheelchair and made a beeline straight toward him. He took a few steps backward, but I kept right on coming. The look on his face changed from one of arrogance to one of panic. He started to flee, and I kept right on coming.

There was no place to go. He slammed into the lockers and turned helplessly toward me with the look in his eyes of someone who was going to pee his pants. I kept charging, pressing my hand as hard as I could onto the throttle. I wanted to hurt him. I wanted to make him pay for all the suffering that he caused everyone. I was out of control. I could not stop.

A crowd soon intervened and the situation began to diffuse. My nurse grabbed my hand and removed it from the controller. She put the wheelchair in reverse and unpinned the bully. Then, she escorted me away as teachers attended to the shocked and embarrassed student.

As my nurse put some distance between us, I felt like shouting back, "Yeah that's right, you just got beat up by a kid in a wheelchair…and I'll do it again, too!"

My heart was pounding. I wanted to go back and finish the job. But my nurse looked me square in the eyes and started to holler.

"Calm down! C.V., calm down right now!"

I had never heard her yell at me like that. That definitely drew my attention away from the bully and onto her. I snapped out of my rage.

"C.V.! C.V.! Stop! C.V.! Listen to me," she said, still in a raised voice. "I know you're upset, but you gotta stop. You can't do this. I don't care if you're right and he's wrong. This is the wrong thing to do. Using your chair like a weapon – it's wrong. You could kill somebody. You gotta stop. You gotta calm down."

She was right and I was embarrassed. Violence was wrong. Violence was what he did…not me. I had to stop. Still, I wondered why it felt right. Why did it feel so good to see a bully finally get put in his place?

The strangest thing about this whole episode is what happened next: nothing. This was a full-fledged fight, in plain sight of many eyewitnesses, and not a single punishment was handed out. And, while it was great not to have this on my permanent record, I wasn't sure that it was for the best intentions. Was it a case of the school officials knowing that it was okay for a bully to be attacked, or was it a case of people not wanting to punish the kid in the wheelchair? If so, then that was definitely NOT what I wanted.

You would think that by now all of my close calls with getting in trouble would have changed my mood and my behavior. Well, you would be wrong. The thought of losing Becca still haunted me. I didn't care about anything else. I continued to act out, not dealing with my newfound feelings in a positive way, but with rebellious and dangerous behavior.

My grades plummeted, but what did I care? Mathematics, one of my best subject, all-of-a-sudden seemed difficult. I couldn't focus on anything, and it didn't matter to me. I felt invisible in that class – like I wasn't getting the attention that I needed. So, I got the notion that if the teacher wanted me to be invisible, well, then that's what I would become.

One morning, I went to school and told the secretary that I had a doctor's appointment from 10:45 to lunchtime (selected to conveniently coincide with math class.) Of course, that was a lie. But what did I care? Nobody would know except for me and my nurse, Debbie, and what could she do? What would she do?

I was right. My nurse did not say a word. Oh, the look on her face told me that I had placed her in an uncomfortable spot (and, in looking back, I do feel bad about that) but she just kept quiet and followed me. She didn't feel it was her place to discipline me, just to keep me and others around me safe.

The secretary gave me the pass, and I strolled right out the front door, smiling with my nurse dutifully by my side. Who knew it could be that easy?

The day was beautifully sunny; and I felt such a feeling of freedom and accomplishment. I felt proud of myself, albeit for the wrong reasons. We walked right past people and no one said a word. Nobody ever questioned what I was doing or why I was not in school. Maybe they thought that if Debbie was with me, I was doing what I was supposed to be doing. Again, I felt wickedly content in knowing what I could get away with.

We strolled out of the school parking lot and headed toward an old barn that was right next to the school. I had always wanted to explore that barn, so I felt like this was as good an opportunity as ever. We walked around it for a while until we came across a large painted turtle. Debbie picked it up and held it close to me to look at. Its shell was so beautiful, yet I laughed every time that it poked its head out of it and then back in when it became scared. I remembered reading about how turtles were one of the few species to survive from way back in the days of the dinosaurs. I admired that because that meant that they were strong.

I asked Debbie if we could keep the turtle, but she told me that there was no way to bring it home. I think she was looking out for me again, because, if you think about it, how was I going to explain returning from the doctor's with a turtle? I guess that if I wanted to continue my evil, school-skipping ways, I had better think things through more thoroughly.

We said goodbye to the turtle and set him free. I still felt bored and restless, so I decided to find something else to do. And, since it just so happens that my church was right across the street from the Junior High School, I decided to pay it a visit. Again I floored the throttle of my wheelchair and took off. Debbie followed. I bet she was nervous.

I quickly made my way toward the parking lot exit so that I could cross the road that separated the church from the school. Debbie followed. I bet she was even more nervous now, as sometimes cars moved pretty fast as they drove on that road. On our way, my chorus teacher, Mrs. C. happened to drive by. She asked me if I was out for my morning stroll. I just smiled, said "Yes," and happily went on my way, not worrying anymore about why it was so easy to get away with things.

At church I said hello to two of my good friends, the church secretary and the pastor. We talked for a while, just the usual chit-chat about what nice weather we were having and was I going to be in church on Sunday. Neither one of them questioned why I was not in school. A pattern was developing. It was amazing. I was invincible.

I said goodbye and headed toward the church kitchen with thoughts of a quick peanut butter and jelly sandwich in my head, but Debbie didn't like that idea. She told me that it was getting close to the time that I had told everyone I would be back. She convinced me that it was time to return. I think she didn't want to see me get into trouble. Neither did I. Getting away with it was just too much fun. So I again revved up my chair and headed out the door, across the road and into school.

Back at school, I realized that I still had a few minutes to spare. What to do next, I wondered? I felt proud of pulling off my caper, so I decided to parade around the school and wave hello to everyone. An achievement like this should be shared with the masses. We walked and waved, walked and waved, until we came to the Math classroom.

Class was still in session, so I decided to brazenly sit right outside the window, at the scene of the crime, in plain view of everyone. It's amazing how fast a criminal can become arrogant. Again I smiled and waved at everyone I saw.

Not wanting to be too cocky – or get caught – I decided that the best course of action was to finish off my day as if nothing irregular had happened at all. And this almost worked. Halfway through the last period of the day, a call came into the classroom. It was the Principal's Office requesting to see me immediately.

On my way down, I didn't feel so proud anymore. I was nervous about what might happen. A major dose of reality had just taken hold of me. I began to get very, very worried. I realized that I was not acting like myself and I had gotten caught. I had no idea what the punishment would be, but thought that nothing could be

121

worse than the feeling I was feeling in the pit of my stomach at that moment.

Debbie immediately saw that I was upset. She once again stepped in to save my butt. (Note: any school officials reading this book are advised to skip to the next chapter.) She told me that if I did not want to get into trouble, I should pretend to cry when I got into the office.

At first, I thought that was a pretty lame idea. I didn't know if I could pull it off and I didn't want to look like an even bigger fool. I remember hearing people say that if you lie about things, you only make them worse, so I figured I had better tell the truth and take my punishment like a man. Still, if a few tears could get me off a little easier, who was I to argue with success? I decided to give it a try.

When I got there, the whole interrogation squad was waiting for me: the principal, the vice principal, and my guidance counselor, who was the first to speak up.

"Craig, did you skip math class today?" she asked, looking disappointed.

"Yes."

"Why?" she asked again.

Before I had a chance to answer her question, I opened the spigot on the water works. Tears started pouring down my face. It was great. I had no idea that I could actually do that. It was almost like I was a professional actor, a Broadway star. I had a feeling that the ploy might work.

Between bursts of tears I opened up to the officials. After all, people did want some kind of an explanation. I told everyone that I was having problems in math class and that I wasn't getting the attention that I needed. I told them that I needed help, but wasn't getting enough from my math teacher. All of this was true. But then I went a bit too far.

"I bet I have your attention now, don't I?" I arrogantly blurted out.

My guidance counselor gave me a dirty look. Realizing that I had pushed my luck to its limit, I shut up.

I never told anyone at school the real reason why I skipped class or had been acting the way that I was. I never admitted it to anyone back then. But I knew. My spiraling behavior was all due to not knowing how to deal with my feelings about losing Becca.

I had learned my lesson about acting out. The feeling of getting in trouble had left a knot in my stomach. I knew I had to change and change soon. I knew I needed to bring my grades back up. I knew that I had to get over losing Becca.

The question was, how?

Chapter Sixteen: A New Challenge

I was thirteen, emotional, and confused – just like every other thirteen-year-old on the planet. My problem was that I couldn't get over my breakup with Becca. So I decided that if I immersed myself in my music, it might help me forget about losing her – well as much as anyone could ever forget losing such a wonderful person. If anything could get me through it, it would be my music. Luckily, the Fulton Community Theater was putting on a performance of "Alice in Wonderland" later that summer, so I motored right down there and signed up. I was on cloud nine.

The theater became my home away from home. The house where I lived was a roof, walls and a floor, but the theater was my escape into a home that existed deep inside me. It was a place where nothing mattered; not appearance, shape, size, color, or even arms and legs; nothing except your voice, your song, the essence of your being. These were my people. I was accepted here. This was where I belonged. Put me in my costume. Show me to the stage. I will walk. I will run. I will fly.

I already knew a lot of the cast members, so when I showed up for the first rehearsal, it was like a reunion of sorts. It didn't matter much what play we did, or what part I got to play, I knew it was going to be fun. I was again asked to do a solo. Even though there are more solos in Community Theater than in chorus, it is still an honor to be chosen to do one, since most of the singing is done by the ensemble cast.

Although I thoroughly enjoyed each and every minute of practice, rehearsal, and performance, I started noticing something disturbing. I started getting the feeling that my voice was starting to go. No one said a word to me, so I figured it was just my imagination, just the fact that I have a keen ear for sound and tended to be a perfectionist as far as music was concerned. I figured that if others still made a big fuss over me, then I must still be fine.

Days passed and I still noticed a struggle singing. At first I thought that perhaps my voice was changing. After all, I had started to grow, so maybe that altered my voice a bit. That might explain why some of the high notes were harder to hit, but it did not explain why I was having trouble breathing during singing, and why it began to hurt to do so. Still, I ignored it and followed the old adage of "The show must go on."

The show did go on as planned and it was a huge success. I reluctantly said goodbye to my friends for the remainder of the summer with thoughts of some quiet time on the beach in my head. But that never happened.

My health started to deteriorate. My breathing became inhibited by something. My whole body felt worse and worse with each passing day. It became harder to get into a comfortable position. It became harder to breathe at all. I was slouched over all the time, looking warped and distorted. The pain kept increasing and it left me puzzled, cranky, and a bit scared.

How could this be? I kept asking myself. *I keep trying. I try to have*

126

positive thoughts. But something always pulls the rug out from under me. What in the world is going on? What in the world is happening to me now? Just when I think I have it all under control. What now? What did I do to deserve this?

My family soon realized that we had another medical problem to deal with. They immediately took me to a doctor to get an opinion as to what was happening and how we could deal with it. The preliminary results were not good. I was diagnosed with scoliosis, a severe curvature of the spine. Because I was growing and gaining weight, this was putting a great amount of pressure on the left side of my body, my weaker side. And it was crushing my left lung. If we did not do something about it, I would die. I would crush myself to death.

The weird thing about this problem was that it was not because of my disease, per se. It was because I was *surviving* the disease. Simply put, because I did not die, my lack of developing muscles and weak skeletal frame could not handle the stress from all the weight that was now being applied to it. My living and growing was killing me from the inside out.

It almost sounds incomprehensible, but my success was now causing my failure. Once again it was time to go into fight mode. Once again it was necessary to do battle if I was going to stay alive.

My mom immediately switched into overdrive. She started doing research online. She started looking for specialists, if there were any at all. She scoured the planet for every imaginable option. If there was anything out there to be found, you can rest assured she would find it. We all had complete faith in her.

It was clear that I needed some sort of procedure that would strengthen my back and take the burden off my lungs. I needed to find a way to be able to sit up straight again. Naturally, I had just assumed that my mother would find a quick and easy solution. But it soon became clear that nothing about this was going to be quick or easy.

"Craig, we need to talk," Mom said to me one evening.

Mom had a look on her face that was not quite as shiny and beautiful as her everyday look. She looked upbeat, but not as much as usual. I could tell immediately that something was up. Whenever someone says "We need to talk," the talk is not usually good.

"I think I have an idea of how to solve your problem."

"OK, Mom, lay it on me. I can take it," I replied.

"Well, I am sorry to say this," she continued, "but I don't think there's any way to fix the problem with your spine without some sort of operation. I think you are going to need surgery."

I didn't like that word one bit. I couldn't face the thought of someone doing that to me. After all that I had been through – the needles and the machines and the medicine and the gadgets and the poundings on my tender skin – after all of that, now they were going to cut me open? No way!

I could face a lot of things, but not that. Not at that moment. I looked the other way and left the room as fast as I could.

I did not say another word about it for a very long time. Mom would say things, try to cheer me up, put a positive spin on it, but I refused to speak. This was more than I could handle. She realized this right away, so she kept right on making plans behind my back. Soon she approached me again with the proposition that I see a specialist in Syracuse, just to get the facts. By that time I was struggling with my breathing so much that I knew there was no other option. I agreed to get help.

Mom must have had a case of déjà vu, because we were repeating all of the steps we went through when I was a baby and on the verge of being diagnosed with SMA. First we head to a local physician. Then to Syracuse for another opinion. Where would the trip take us this time?

The specialist from Syracuse did not paint a pretty picture. While he did say that there was a procedure that might fix the problem, that procedure was intense, to say the least. It involved having a rod surgically placed in my back from the base of my neck all the way down to my hips. This rod would be attached inside me and would make it possible for me to sit straight. The problem is that to do the surgery, I would have to be put on a ventilator. Then the doctor came right out and admitted that if I survived the long, complicated surgery, there was still only a thirty percent chance that I would ever come off the ventilator. Ever.

Again, I could not say a word. I sat there in shock as people debated what to do with my life. Again I felt vulnerable. Again I felt helpless. After all my hard work – after all the years – I was back to this.

My mind began to picture the future. There I was, sitting tall and strong in my chair...with a ventilator tube coming out of me. There would be no talking. There would be no singing. My music would be dead. And as far as I was concerned, I would just as soon join it.

Although I never spoke my mind, somehow my mother read it. I was never happier than when I heard her decision of what to do.

"Thirty percent? Nope. No way," she told the doctor. "That's not good enough. I do not want my son on a ventilator for the rest of his life! We will look for another solution. There has *got* to be another solution. We will not give up until we find it."

And she didn't. Mom tirelessly searched, never letting the idea that this might be the end of the line for me enter into her head. But I have to admit that it did enter mine. I could not get the thought out of my head. Mom kept repeating over and over that it was all a case of the odds. If one doctor thought I had a thirty percent chance of making it, well, then, maybe the next doctor would say fifty percent, or seventy percent. Who knew?

Finally, Mom had a breakthrough. She read something about this doctor in New Jersey who was a specialist in dealing with kids with Spinal Muscular Atrophy Type 1. That alone gave us cause to have hope. His name was Dr. Bach, and he was making a name for himself by using innovative procedures. And when Mom saw his picture on the cover of a magazine, that did it. Right then and there a trip to New Jersey was planned.

I did not want to make the trip. Newark, New Jersey seemed light-years away from comfortable old Fulton, New York. The thought of being cooped up and uncomfortable in my van for eight or nine hours did not appeal to me one bit. I would much rather have been lounging on a beach listening to some music or racing around town trying to create a breeze on my face by going as fast as I could. Going to see yet another doctor was not my idea of fun. It seemed like another agony that I would have to endure.

Endure it is just what I did. In what seemed like the blink of an eye we were face to face with Dr. Bach. And although I was rapidly becoming skeptical, I found him to be a different sort of doctor. He had a strong voice and a friendly look of confidence: dark brown hair and a tiny smile that made you feel like you were in competent hands. It was like he was saying "I know what I am doing, so if you want to succeed you better follow me." I liked that feeling. I liked it a lot.

Dr. Bach and his whole respiratory team thoroughly

examined me, something which by then was as common and boring to me as brushing my teeth, if only I could do that. He told us that I was a remarkable case, I was doing amazingly well for someone with my condition, and that he would like to work with me. It all sounded so wonderfully positive for a change. Then, he introduced me to a whole new arsenal of equipment that I would have to start using every day if I were to stay alive.

My first new mechanical "buddy" was the Cough Assist. The Cough Assist was a face mask and hose that attached tightly over my mouth and nose. The opposite end connected to a machine that produced positive and negative air pressure. The principle behind its operation was to push air into the chest and then pull it out. Its goal was to keep the lungs clear. Everyone knew right away that this machine was intended for me. I had such trouble coughing and my inability to do so was always causing me to come down with pneumonia.

Although the Cough Assist worked fine, using it was no picnic. In order for it to work, it had to "take over." By this I mean that, when someone flipped its switch, it began doing all my breathing for me. It was impossible to draw in a breath when the machine was sucking all the air out of me and, likewise it was impossible to exhale while it was pushing air into my lungs. It's a pretty scary feeling because I had to completely surrender to a machine. At first, my body fought it because it's an unnatural feeling. But then I relaxed and my mind calmed down because I knew that was saving my life. I would need to do this every single day, as long as I live.

Next up was something called the Therabite. This is more like a tool than a machine. It is fairly small, mostly plastic, and has hinged parts. The Therabite (today known as the Ora-Stretch) is designed to strengthen the muscles in your mouth and jaw area. It is placed with one end inside the mouth and the other sticking out of it. Then someone presses up and down several times, forcing the mouth to open wide. If I did not do this, I would slowly lose my mouth muscles and my mouth would become unable to open on its own. And if that happened, there would be no way to eat regular food.

That is pretty scary if you think about it. So I try not to think about it. I also try not to think about all the kids who went before me and did not have these tools. All the kids that did not make it for one reason or another. I try not to think about them because it would be overwhelming. What I do try to think about is what I can do to get better; and how maybe my struggles and pain will help some other kid along the way.

Everyone was impressed with Dr. Bach. With every word he said, I kept hearing this voice inside my head saying "Finally! Someone who knows about me. Someone who knows my disease. Someone who has positive ideas. Someone who can give me hope."

Dr. Bach was also optimistic about the possibility of me having back surgery. The difference between him and other doctors was that he was against putting SMA patients on ventilators unless it was the last resort. I remember him saying something about "no-traching," which meant that he would not do as the other doctors had suggested and put me on a ventilator strictly as a knee-jerk reaction. He believed the airway should be kept clear and unencumbered. Everyone remembered how the first doctor had said that the chance of ever coming off a ventilator was low, so this was wonderful to hear. Still, big decisions had to be made.

After our visit with Dr. Bach, we went to see another doctor, the surgeon who would do the operation itself – if that is what we decided to do. He was also very optimistic about not using a ventilator. The only problem was that he warned us all that the chance of surviving the operation was not as high as we had thought.

132

No matter what we decided to do, high risk was involved. So we were sent home with a Cough Assist, a Therabite, and a huge decision to make.

My life lay in the balance.

Chapter Seventeen: Tough Decisions

The trip home seemed twice as long as the trip to see Dr. Bach. No one wanted to talk about our experiences in Newark. It was too much to handle. We were tired of hearing about machines and procedures, surgeries and ventilators. There was no way to make sense out of it, or to decide which thing to do without experiencing a flood of mixed feelings. We rode along in silence as the tall buildings slowly changed into smaller and smaller ones and the browns and grays of the city changed into the muted greens of the mountains.

When the conversation finally started, I plainly stated to Mom that I did not want to have the surgery and that I was fine the way I was. I was trying to put on a brave face, but I wasn't fooling anyone. The fact of the matter was that I was not fine the way I was. I knew it. Everyone knew it. My condition was going to kill me if something was not done. If I decided not to have the operation, I would keep growing and crush myself to death on the inside. If I decided to take a chance and go under the knife, there was a good chance that I would either die, become a vegetable, or live out the rest of my days constantly hooked up to a machine. Some choices.

As we got closer to home, I looked out of the window and

watched my world return. I needed the comfort of familiar surroundings to wash the confusion that tugged away at my insides. I needed to get away from all that. Maybe at home I would have time to escape and think things through. Maybe that's all that I would need. Exhausted, confused, and unclear about my future, I dropped off to sleep.

The next days of my summer were uncomfortable, to say the least. We spent a lot of time arguing and debating and going over options. I knew that Mom wanted me to have the surgery done. She was very clear about that. She felt it was the only way to improve my life. Looking back, she was right. If I wanted any chance at being able to sit up, talk, sing – things that I had become used to doing – I had to roll the dice. But I didn't see it that way. In my mind, it was either die one way or die the other way. I could not see a successful outcome to this battle. It was going to take a lot of arm twisting to get me to see things Mom's way.

My grandparents felt that we should leave it up to God to decide. I didn't understand what that meant. I couldn't imagine that if we asked God a question, we'd really get an answer. God doesn't make phone calls or send emails. How could He answer us? How could He tell us what to do? It made no sense to me. Still, Grandma and Grandpa felt that we should pray about it, and I figured, what harm could it do? So we all prayed and waited for an answer.

One Sunday at church, Grandma sped things up by going public. She made her way to the microphone at the pulpit during a time when people make announcements. I wasn't sure what she was up to. She always did a lot of work on fundraisers and helping to get food donated to feed the hungry, but she hadn't been working on anything like that for a while. I had no idea what she was going to talk about. Then, in a simple, straightforward way, she spoke.

"I would like to ask everyone to pray for C.V. He is very ill

136

right now. We just took a trip to see some doctors in New Jersey, and they told us about a back operation he could have that might save his life. It's very risky. He might not survive it. We are confused about what to do, so please keep our whole family in your prayers. Thank you."

Grandma went back and took her place in the choir. Not another word was said. The church was very quiet for a while. I could feel everyone staring at me. I could see people wiping tears from their eyes. I was embarrassed. I was uncomfortable. Finally, the pastor spoke, worship service began and things got back to normal.

After church service, I was still feeling embarrassed, so I decided to make a fast dash for the Fellowship Hall, where they always had an outrageously delicious array of cookies, cakes and assorted snacks to go along with coffee, tea and other drinks. At least if I could drown my frustration in some sugar and caffeine, I might feel a little better for a while. Besides, at that point, I really didn't feel like hanging out with Grandma, since I knew that everyone in the church would be seeking her out with a million personal questions about the operation.

Grandma eventually caught up to me, along with everybody else in the church, and sure enough they had questions. Dozens upon dozens of them. And they offered well-wishes, which seemed like hundreds. I felt on the spot and uncomfortable again. I was used to being the center of attention from time to time, but it was usually for doing something good. Not for this. I didn't like this. This felt like pity, even though I knew it wasn't. I knew it was just people offering help and support. It was just people doing the right thing.

Most of the people were familiar to me. After all, I had grown up in the church. Everybody knew me and I recognized most of them as well. But one face was different. There was one person who was a stranger.

He introduced himself as "Lou." He told us that he was a police officer for the Port Authority of New York and New Jersey. He was just in town for a few days for a 25th wedding anniversary party of friends of our family. He said that he was often stationed at Newark Airport, and that he knew the area very well. Then he told us that he wanted to offer us help if we decided to have the operation. He was a very friendly guy and seemed nice, so we exchanged email addresses and left it at that, since we still hadn't decided what to do.

Summer was drawing to an end. Decision time was approaching, but I tried putting it off as much as possible. I hated talking about anything to do with it; it was always in the back of my head. I kept wondering how many days I had left to live. Every night when I went to bed, I couldn't help but wonder if I would wake up the next morning. Even though I tried to keep distracted and I never talked about it to anyone, it consumed me.

Mom knew the time had come to put her foot down, so one day she took me to an ice cream stand by the lake. It was there that she told me that she decided to go through with the surgery.

"Craig, I know that you're not going to like this," she began.

By that time I already knew what she was going to say. It didn't take a genius to figure it out.

"You're not getting any better, and I hate to see you suffer like this. I have decided to go through with the surgery."

I felt like hollering. I felt like saying "*You* decided? *You?* What about me? Don't I get a say in this? It's my life. Doesn't what I want count?"

But I didn't. I didn't say a thing. I just looked at Mom. Tears were running down her cheeks. It was then that I realized that this was just as hard for her as it was for me. If I died, it didn't just mean that I would lose the person closest to me in life. It would mean that we *both* would. And it was still way too soon to let that happen. I was worried and scared, but I knew that it was probably for the best.

"Okay, Mom," was all I said.

We tried our best to maintain our lives as if things were as normal as ever, even though surgery day was looming ahead. Mom kept busy by contacting doctors and setting everything up. I kept busy by focusing on the start of a brand new school year.

A few weeks later, I began the 8th grade. I was on the Green Team this year and trying to get excited about it, but it was just no use. My mind was someplace else, far, far away. I was frightened and unfocused, plus Becca wasn't with me, and the sadness of losing her still lingered in my heart. I felt out of place just being at school. It felt temporary. I didn't know where I belonged anymore. Life felt more fragile than ever.

Soon word spread about my impending surgery and I was flooded with attention. Again a lot of it felt like pity and that left me with a bad taste in my mouth. I tried to be polite and go along with it, keep quiet and just say "thank you," but inside I was churning with uneasiness. The only good thing – if it was a good thing – was that my surgery was set for about two weeks from the start of school. That was plenty of time to do battle with the emotions of the situation before I would have to deal with the even tougher, physical challenge.

Just before I left school – for a prolonged period or forever, no one knew – one of my teachers presented me with a framed picture of the entire 8th grade Green Team and said "We are all behind you, Craig," which meant so much to me. I left school that day with tears in my eyes and fear in my heart. Right after that, Becca stopped by to wish me good luck. She looked a bit frightened and it made me wonder if she was thinking this would be the last time she ever saw me. The same thought ran through my mind. Would I ever see her beautiful face again?

My family was almost as scared as I was. Our lives were going to be turned upside down for the 18 billionth time. We had no idea of how long we would have to stay down there in "the big city," a place so unlike Fulton. Newark, New Jersey intimidated everyone. It scared us so much that my grandma decided to take Lou up on his offer. She emailed him and told him of our plans. In no time at all, he made good on his word. In no time at all, we were overwhelmed by the kindness and generosity of the people he knew.

Just before we left, a friend of Lou's who was a baggage supervisor at the airport, offered to try and find a private plane to fly us to Newark. That didn't work out because I would have had to sit in my wheelchair in the plane, which wasn't safe. Still, we were amazed at the kindness of the offer.

The generosity didn't end there. Lou told us he was contacting hotels near the hospital, trying to find us a decent place to stay. He felt that this was important, as it might help my family relax at the end of a long and stressful day at the hospital. He talked to the manager of a new Marriott Fairfield Hotel and told him my story. The manager agreed to give us a reduced rate on a beautiful room for an extended stay. The hotel was less than ten minutes from the hospital, which made it convenient for everyone. It was also right across from the Statue of Liberty. Many times during our stay there, I stared at it for a long time, until my mind was someplace else and I started to relax again.

Although we left for New Jersey on a Thursday, my surgery wasn't scheduled until the following Monday. The only thing scheduled in between was to visit the anesthesiologist. That left us with a lot of time on our hands to sit and think and become more nervous and scared. I couldn't help but wonder how they were going to put support rods in my back and how that would feel. I couldn't get the doctor's words out of my head, especially when he talked about the danger of working so close to the spinal cord and the huge risk of infection because of how long the operation would take and how much they had to cut me open. My skin was absolutely crawling with uneasiness and a biting feeling of impending doom washed over me like an icy shower. I was afraid that I was going to die. I just wanted to go home. I just wanted to go back to when I was small and everything seemed easier. I could see no future.

Once again, downstate generosity came to my rescue.

We got a phone call from Lou, and he told us that one of his supervisors at the Port Authority had given him permission to borrow a transportation minibus with a safety wheelchair lift, so he could drive us around the city. We were thrilled because, even though we were told the trip to the hospital was only ten minutes, it could have been on Mars for all we knew about how to get around the area. Lou also told us that he would be stopping by to show us around and help us get used to the neighborhood. Of course we said "yes" immediately.

When he got to our hotel, not only did Lou have the minibus, but he also had presents for me! One of his co-workers had given him a baseball that was signed by New York Yankees manager Joe Torre. He told him to give it to me. The equipment manager of the New York Giants gave him a football that the team had used in their last game and told Lou to "Give it to the kid. We hope it brings him good luck!" I wasn't sure if I believed in luck, in signs, or anything like that; but if there ever was a time to think they did exist, now was as good a time as any for me to start.

I later came to find out that, being a Port Authority Police Officer, Lou lost many of his friends and co-workers on September

141

11th. I also learned that he was involved in the dreadful clean-up effort that followed and was still going on. And I learned that many of the people who were now helping me out had the exact same story to tell. And yet, they were taking time out to help me. This meant more to me than I can ever say.

Lou drove us all over town. First, he showed us how to get to the hospital so we would be comfortable making the trip when we had to do it alone. Then he showed us the sights. He showed us what parts of town were "good parts" and what parts we should avoid. That made us feel a little nervous again, but better to be safe than sorry.

Although Lou did a lot to help us feel better, pass the time, and even have a little fun, we all knew that reality would sink in again very soon. Whenever we were alone at our hotel, the situation was tense. I knew everyone was nervous, but nobody really said a word about it. I had the feeling that they didn't want to let me see them like that. I had a feeling that my family just felt like sitting close to me, as calm and as quiet as possible, with forced smiles on their faces to cheer me up. I got the feeling that we all knew I was going to die.

Right before surgery day, I had a weird dream. It was vivid, yet I never figured out what it meant. I dreamt I was flying around. My arms were like wings, moving and flapping, yet I could not feel them. I jetted past the Statue of Liberty and she waved her torch at me and smiled. I flew into New York City and saw even bigger buildings that seemed to pierce the sky. I flew over Yankee Stadium and the whole team came onto the field and waved to me. It made no sense at all, but it made me feel happy.

When I awoke, I remembered the dream. I thought about it, trying to figure out its meaning. Did it mean I would have my disease cured? But that was impossible. Or maybe it meant I was going to die. Maybe everyone was saying goodbye to me. Maybe I was flying up to Heaven. If that's what it meant, if that's what it felt like to be dead, I thought, then it wasn't that bad after all. Maybe I shouldn't be scared. But that feeling of calm did not last very long.

Monday morning came.

Lou showed up bright and early the day of the surgery. He told us to leave everything up to him and that he would drive us all to the hospital. The trip there was awkward. No one wanted to speak. We were all too nervous, so we just let Lou do the talking and sat there quietly.

I tried to put the negative thoughts out of my head, but it was impossible. Until that time, I had always thought of myself as a positive person. But this time it was hard to feel that way. It was hard to forget the facts and focus on a positive outcome without having all the dangers pop into my head. I could not help but think about how I was going to be cut open, my whole back from my neck to my tail bone just cut right open. I felt like I was about to be butchered just like an animal. I was so scared.

I was in the pre-op room with my family, when four or five doctors came in to see me. They had markers in their hands and told me they had to make marks on my back for surgery. They began drawing on my back, and I became even more afraid. Now it became all too real. Now I could feel *where* they were going to cut me. I felt like crying because I knew that within an hour, I would be going under the knife. And sure enough, about an hour later, the doctors came back. It was time to go.

They let me say my goodbyes to my family. One by one they came up to me. Everyone was crying. Everyone tried to say something, but the words always got choked up in their throats. It didn't matter. I knew what they meant. Finally, it was time for my mom to say goodbye.

I had always been scared to have the operation; but by now my fear had turned to panic.

"I have got to get out of this," I thought, *"I don't want this. I have to get out of here. I can't do this."*

Mom started talking to me, but I could not hear her words.

"I don't want the surgery anymore, Mom," I said. "I changed my mind."

"Shhh," she answered, "Everything is going to be fine."

How could it be fine? How could it? I was going to die! I was sure of it. I saw the signs and they all told me I was going to die. Please, somebody let me go home. Please, somebody get me out of here. I don't want to do this!

"No, Mom, I can't. I can't do this!"

"Oh, Craig, you can do this," she said, tears now streaming down her cheeks.

"No, Mom, I can't. I can't do it. I'm gonna die!"

They kept pushing the stretcher closer and closer to the operating room. Mom was walking right beside me, holding onto my hand. The lights in the corridor seemed to be going by faster and faster and my heart felt like it was going to jump out of my chest.

"Baby, you're not going to die."

I looked into her eyes. She was sobbing and having a hard time speaking.

"You're not going anywhere. It's not your time. I just know it. God has a plan for you. You are not supposed to die here. There are bigger and better things ahead in your life, Honey. You're not going to die today."

We were right outside the operating room. The doctors stopped us and told Mom that she could not go inside. This was it. Mom leaned down and kissed me.

"I love you, Craig."

But all I could think about was leaving.

"No, please! Please! I want to go home! Please!"

They opened the doors and wheeled me into the room. I couldn't see my mother anymore.

With all my might I yelled to her, "Mommy, I love you!"

Chapter Eighteen: The Operation

It was the brightest place I had ever been in, brighter than the blazing sun at Fair Haven Beach in the dog days of August, brighter than the four-foot banks of snow that sprang up in Fulton's never-ending winter season, making the whole town seem like one giant bobsled course. It was the intense brightness of the operating room. The ceiling was a sea of lights: big ones, little ones, and emergency ones in case those failed.

With all the bright lights and glow surrounding me, I began to wonder if it was a dream, if I was dead or if I had been slipped some hallucinogenic drugs. And since, to my knowledge, no one had yet given me anything, I started wondering if this was Heaven. I soon found out. Everyone began poking me and prodding me, moving my fragile limbs this way and that. I knew then that I could not have been in Heaven unless all the stories about the place were amazingly inaccurate.

Strange masked faces bobbed into view for a split second and then disappeared from sight. I could not make out who they were, since the glare from the lights filled the room with a silvery haze. A few of the masked faces said "Hello" or "Hi" or "Relax, Craig." But that was not possible, unless of course they could find a way to confuse me into a stupor. And, boy did they try.

The room was buzzing with activity, and I tried in vain to follow the images of the people that darted past me. It was impossible to focus on anyone for more than a second or two. I was cold. The room was cold. Everything was cold but the lights.

Someone grabbed my arm. Then a leg. They moved me this way and that. I felt like a science project. Once in a while, someone would ask, "How ya doin?", but I couldn't reply. I was numb with fear.

I could hear voices in my head. I could hear Grandma telling me that I was strong and could handle whatever came my way and Grandpa telling me to get better fast so we could sing together again. I could hear my stepdad telling me how proud he was to have me as his son and Cralynne telling me to hurry home because she had just bought a great new CD of a band she thought I would like. I could hear my pastor and the people from church again; and I remembered how they called me just to wish me good luck. And I heard Mom's voice telling me how much she loved me. All these voices were real and powerful. All these voices gave me strength. I wasn't afraid anymore.

I heard the slow *beep, beep, beep* of the machines, so I knew that they were monitoring my heart and my breathing and my life. At that moment, time stopped. A doctor placed a mask over my face, and told me to count to ten. I almost laughed when I heard that because it seemed so unreal to me. I remembered seeing this scene in every medical show on television or in the movies. I always wondered how accurate it was. It seemed impossible for any drug to act that fast. I hoped and I prayed that it did and it wasn't just Hollywood magic, because there was no way that I wanted to be even a tiny bit conscious when they started the cutting. No way on earth.

My breathing was shallow, and I felt weak as I began to count.

"One…two…"

This may sound crazy, and for all I know it may be a dream, but just at that moment I started to float in the room right above everyone. I saw myself on the operating table as they prepared me for surgery. I saw the doctor leaning over me, pressing the mask over my nose and mouth. I could see someone else wheeling in a tray of shiny silver operating tools and another person turning some dials on a machine.

"Three…"

Three. I distinctly remember getting to three. After that, everything went totally black. There's nothing else I remember. Not the counting. Not the dream. Not the surgery.

As anyone who has ever gone under the knife will tell you, it is a blessing to be able to say that you can't remember a single thing about the procedure. I agree. I am happy to say that the only things I know about what happened are the things that others have told me. I do not recall being cut open or getting blood transfusions. The support rods were placed inside me and attached to my skeletal system in several places without me seeing or feeling a thing. I am extremely grateful that I was out cold the entire time.

The operation lasted eleven and a half hours, plus two more to get more than 400 stitches put in. There were 200 stitches inside me and over 200 stitches on the outside holding me together. It was done. I survived.

I woke up about 22 hours after surgery, or so they tell me. By that time, I was so out of it that you could have told me I was the president of the United States and I would have believed you. All I can remember for a while after that was pain. So much pain.

Slowly the faded edges that divided my dream world from my waking world grew stronger and more pronounced. I was starting to come out of the daze. Or was I? I heard voices, women's voices, and they were singing.

There by my bedside was my mother. Alongside of her was my older cousin who lived in Pennsylvania. She had driven in to see how I was doing. And now, the two of them were singing me back to life.

I wanted to smile but I couldn't. My mouth hurt. Something uncomfortable was in my mouth. I could hardly open it at all. I was confused. I didn't know what was going on. When I started to moan, a nurse quickly came over to me. She could tell what was bothering me and she tried to calm me down.

"Don't worry, Craig," she said. "I know it feels uncomfortable, but that's just the intubation tube. You are on a ventilator to help you breath."

I wanted to scream "No! This wasn't supposed to happen!" but that only made it harder to breathe.

"What's going on?" I thought. *"He promised he wouldn't put me on a ventilator! No, this can't be. He promised!"*

Thoughts of all the pre-operation facts and figures ran through my head at once. I was doomed. The operation may have been a success, but I was doomed. I would have to join all those others who remained on a ventilator for the rest of their lives.

Panicked, I looked straight at Mom. I tried to shake my head "no" but it was no use. I couldn't move. Again I moaned and tried to speak. Tears welled up in my eyes. Mom knew immediately what the matter was.

"Shhhh, shhh," she said sweetly and with a smile. "It's fine. Everything is fine. The ventilator is just temporary. The doctor promised to take it out soon. He said your breathing was good, remarkably good. He said that they will take out the tube soon. You won't have to stay like this."

Her words were music to my ears, and almost as sweet as the voices that awakened me; but that just wasn't good enough for me. No, it had to be better than that. I had to do better. So I choked and strained and mumbled out a few words.

"Oh, now, please don't try to speak," Mom said. "It's impossible. You won't be able to speak until the tube comes out."

"No good," I thought. *"I'm going to speak and that is that!"*

Again I tried to get a sentence out. This time the nurse saw me and tried to stop me, too.

"Craig, please calm down," she said. "You're only going to hurt yourself. People can't talk when they are intubated."

In one ear and out the other. When I want to do something, I am going to do it.

"Hi, Mom," I said.

Her eyes widened and got teary. The nurse put her hand over her mouth to hide her amazement.

"Hi, Mom."

"Hi. How are you feeling?"

"It hurts."

151

"I know, Honey. I know. It's going to hurt for a while. They have medicine to give you when it gets bad. It will get better soon. I promise, OK?"

"OK, Mom," I answered.

Everyone could not believe what was happening. The doctors had said that it would be physically impossible for me to talk while I was on a ventilator. The only problem is that the doctors didn't know me well enough. They didn't know how many times I had beaten the odds. But I did.

At that point, just about everything came back into focus. My back hurt so much, and I was dog-tired, but I was alive. I was alive. Over and over, I kept telling myself, *"I am alive!"*

Chapter Nineteen: Recovery

To say that I was in a good mood after the operation would be like saying that the sky is just something that holds the air we breathe. Just opening my eyes and seeing the light of day made me smile. I am almost ashamed to admit it, but I thought the operation was the end of the line for me. I had doubts whether or not I would survive the surgery. But everything worked: the procedure, the prayers. Everything. And even with that dumb old tube in my mouth, I still think people could tell I was smiling.

I was giddy. Everything seemed to make me laugh. When the doctor explained that the 12-hour surgery to correct my scoliosis and implant the rod in my back had actually made me four inches taller, it was all that I could do to stop myself from bursting out in laughter. All kinds of silly thoughts ran through my head.

I wonder if I will still fit in my wheelchair. Maybe I will need bigger pants. I heard they were having a sale at Barney's. Maybe we can stop there on the way home. If I practice my lay-ups, I wonder if the Knicks would give me a tryout. You get the idea. I was completely loopy – that is until the drugs started wearing off.

It didn't take long to realize that just opening my eyes wasn't good enough. I had a long road ahead of me. There was a high risk that I could get an infection or develop pneumonia. Either one could kill me. I gathered my courage and determination – and sense of humor – and carried on as usual.

I was hooked up to every machine imaginable. I had a ventilator to help me breathe, a drainage tube coming out of my back, an intravenous tube to feed me and administer pain and other medications, and a few odds and ends wired to measure my pulse and heart. I think they wanted to hook me up to cable TV, too, but that cost $10 more per day, so we nixed that idea.

Luckily, I was only on the ventilator for two days. The process of getting off it was a bit uncomfortable, but well worth it. Before they could take the tube out, they had to make sure I was going to breathe on my own, so the first step was to turn off the machine and nervously wait. If I couldn't draw a breath and exhale it, then the switch got flipped again and I'd have to wait. If I did breathe, then they could pull the tube out after that, which they did. The doctor smiled and said something about "amazing lung power." That was fine by me. I was free! Now I could really talk…and eat! The only thing left to do was to use the Cough Assist over and over. If that worked, no pneumonia!

After the tubes started coming out, they were able to move me around more and more. This was a pretty scary feeling because you never know what to expect. You are already in pain and frightened that it will increase. You also wonder if you will pop a stitch; but when you have over 400 of them, I guess one or two don't make a big difference.

One of the first things they wanted to see was how I would manage back in my chair again. This was a major hurdle that I would have to jump. Sometime around the third day after surgery I was put to the test. A nurse moved me this way and that. I remember that there didn't seem to be any extra pain from the surgery, only that I could feel something different inside me. The sitting up did not hurt me, but the bending did. I was stiff and uncomfortable and awkward. The doctors said that it was from the rod and that, over time, I would get used to it and hardly notice it at all.

When I was finally able to get into my chair comfortably, and they let me ride around on my own, I fought the urge to go crazy. After all, this was a hospital and there just might be a sick person or two roaming the halls. There was no need to do a wheelie or knock anyone over. I could do all that after I got home.

My stay in the hospital lasted exactly seven days past the day of my surgery. I had passed my tests and I was ready to go home. Boy, was I ready to go home!

Home. I was going home again. Home to my family and friends. Home to my room with my comfortable bed in the corner, just the way I liked it. Home to all my stuff, my TV, and my music. I was going home.

I wasn't the only one getting excited. I could hear it in everyone's voices. In the beginning of the trip, I noticed more of a sense of relief and accomplishment after completing a hard task than anything else. But as we got closer to Fulton, things changed. Now this part of the trip was filled with excitement and anticipation.

"Syracuse!" my stepdad said, as he made it his job to announce our location every few minutes. This made everyone even antsier, because now we knew we were getting close. In about a half hour we would be home.

"It won't be long now!" he said.

I was going nuts. My own music. My own bed. I could just

feel that comfy pillow against my head as the words left his lips. I couldn't wait 30 more minutes. If only I could drive the van. I bet I could get us home in 15.

"Fulton!" he announced, causing everyone to sit up straight. At that point I was beside myself. I almost felt like I could sit up on my own, too.

As the van pulled off of Oneida Street and onto Eighth, everyone shouted at once, "We're home!" By that time I was so crazy excited that I thought I'd pop a stitch.

"Lemme see! Lemme see!" I shouted. "I wanna see our house!"

"Keeps your pants on, Kiddo," said my stepdad. "Let me pull into the driveway first."

The van came to a halt and everyone else got out.

"Me too! Me too!"

"Don't worry," chuckled Mom, "We weren't planning on leaving you in the van."

I tried to laugh, but I didn't find anything funny at that point. I just wanted to get back to my normal world again. Nothing else mattered much.

They lifted me out of my spot and positioned me in my chair. I cringed in pain, but forgot all about that as soon as my eyes saw the house. Our house. So beautiful.

Grandpa opened the front door, and Cralynne shot out past him, running as fast as she could toward us with a huge smile on her face.

"C.V.!" she shouted as she got closer.

I backed my wheelchair off the lift and she pounced on me, giving me the biggest hug of all time. Again I cringed from the pain, but never told anyone because the hug felt a million times better and completely washed it away.

"Hey, don't I get a hug?" kidded my mother.

"In a second," Cralynne answered, knowing that her big brother was finally home. She gave me a second squeeze, this one even harder than the first.

Looks like someone missed me, I thought. *I wonder if I should admit how much I missed her, too. Nah. I still like to keep the upper hand.*

"Hey, C.V.," she said, "I got you something."

Oh, cool, I thought. *A present. I love presents. Maybe everybody will get me a present.*

"What is it?" I asked, knowing that I could not wait another five minutes to get into the house.

"A clean room!" she said, sticking out her tongue at me.

So much for having the upper hand, I thought.

"You didn't touch anything, did you?" I asked.

"Nope. Just kidding."

Seems like someone grew up while I was away, I thought.

While everyone unloaded the van, I made a dash for the door that opened to my room. Cralynne, still glued to my side, opened it, and I flew inside. I looked around, let out a deep breath, and smiled the biggest smile. That night, I devoured a huge supper, after which I slept a most pleasant and contented sleep.

I awoke the next morning to the grim realization that my ordeal was not over yet. I had a lot of pain – the most since leaving the hospital – and I began to see that my rehabilitation would not come at the snap of someone's fingers. It was going to take time and lots of hard work.

The doctor had warned me about all the pain that I would be in, but I had put that completely out of my mind. However, what I felt at that time told me that it was clear he was right on the mark. The first thing I would have to do would be to get medicine into me. Nothing else would be possible without it.

The next thing I had to do was become comfortable with all my new machines and the routine I would have to go through to keep healthy, not just to avoid post-surgery pneumonia, but for the rest of my life. This would prove to be uncomfortable, but worthwhile, to say the least.

The first few weeks home were devoted to getting healthy. There was no talk of going back to school or even going out of the house much. The only place I went was to see a doctor. I got restless. Being home bored me to death. I was alone way too much for my tastes since everyone else was in school. I needed to see my friends more. Oh sure, I could watch as much television as I wanted, but who wanted to? I needed more than television. I could always rely on listening to Metallica to relax me when I felt particularly antsy. But sometimes the family didn't appreciate that, not at the volume that I like to play it. I needed more, and I needed it now.

Unfortunately, I got more, but it wasn't exactly what I had hoped for. Toward the end of October, I got the green light from the doctors. I could now have tutors come in to bring me my school work. Whoopee. I made up my mind that homework was better than nothing. I did my work because there was no way that I wanted to fall so far behind that I had to be held back. I would lose my friends, and that didn't sit right with me. So, I accepted this new reality and plowed right into my schoolwork, just as ferociously as I did everything else.

Sometime in late October the first tutor showed up. It was now time to face another challenge and get back on track. I won't lie and say that I welcomed my tutors with open arms. I didn't look forward to the prospect of doing all that extra work, but I knew it was necessary if I was to have any chance of catching up with my friends and getting my normal life back. And I so desperately wanted that.

"Craig, we have a long road ahead of us. You missed almost two months' worth of school," my tutor explained, as if I really needed that slap in the face.

"Yeah, I know," I answered unexcitedly.

"So when do you want to go back to school?"

"Tomorrow," I answered, knowing that even though it was unrealistic, it was true. I got a semi-nasty look for that.

"No, I mean when do you expect to go back to school? What do the doctors say?"

"The doctors have said maybe after Christmas. But I say *definitely* after Christmas, if not sooner. I want to go back as soon as possible."

"So that's the goal then: after Christmas?"

"Yeah, I guess so."

"Then we have about two months to cover four months of

work," she said.

I really wished she hadn't put it that way. That seemed like a tall mountain to climb. It felt like only yesterday that I had the surgery. Then came the difficult recovery. And now this. Now I would have to work twice as hard as everybody else.

So what's new, I thought. *I always have to work twice as hard as everybody else…or more. I can handle it.*

By Christmas I had caught up to everyone. Now all that I needed was an OK from the doctor and I was all set to resume school in the new year. And that happened, too. I was doing well physically and excited about going back to school. I was going to be able to hang out with my friends, have lunch with my buddies, check out the girls, and talk to everyone imaginable. Life was good.

There was still one thing that worried me a little about returning to school, and that was the inevitable questions that I would have to face. Just about everyone in town had heard about my surgery – and people did a good job about keeping others informed about what was going on – but this was different. This was the unrelenting face-to-face hammering of questions that I dreaded. This was the non-stop, "How did it feel?" "Did it hurt?" "Do you really have a rod inside you?" that I feared. I dreaded having to answer these questions because I thought they might cause me to re-live the ordeal, and, at that point, I wanted nothing more than to move forward, not backwards. I wanted my life back. I wanted to move on.

But soon I found out that questions can be a good thing. They can elevate you from being well-known to rock star status, depending upon how you answer them.

"Dude, did they really cut you wide open?" someone would ask.

"Yup. Wide open. From my neck to my tail bone. Wide open," I'd say. Then I would smile. That would either leave them stunned or completely grossed out.

"Do you really have a rod in you?" I would get asked every fifteen minutes or so.

"Yes, I do. Solid titanium. Stronger than steel." Then I would chuckle a bit and wait for the reaction.

"Did it hurt?" everyone on the face of the earth would ask me.

"Nope. Not at all. Didn't bother me one bit."

That always earned me the most awe. And even though I knew it wasn't true at all, it was fun to say because it wasn't what people expected. Plus, I think it helped me cope with being bombarded with surgery questions. Luckily, after a while, the questions died down and I was allowed to be plain old C.V. And that was fine with me.

A few of my teachers were skeptical when I had told them that I had done all my work, and that I was completely caught up to my classmates in every way. But a few quizzes and questions soon showed them that they should not have doubted me. I had absolutely no trouble at all resuming my studies alongside everyone else, at the same spot, at the same level, and at the same pace. And I was very proud of this achievement. I was back.

I was so happy to be able to blend back in almost immediately. I didn't want anyone to hold me back, or even worse, allow me to pass through out of pity. I wanted exactly what I deserved. I had earned it. Nothing more. Nothing less. I was also allowed to go back to chorus and sing, and I cannot tell you how wonderful that felt to me. I had my music back and that was bliss.

The rest of the school year was uneventful except for one thing. I still missed Becca. We would bump into each other from time to time, which would brighten my day immensely. Those times still felt magical to me. She was always polite and friendly to me, always asked me how I was or if I was seeing anyone. But I wasn't. I hadn't thought about dating in a long time. I was just to the point where I was almost getting over losing her…almost.

School ended and I relished the idea of doing nothing more than relaxing and having fun. I was glad junior high school was over. I had lost my girlfriend and endured a horrible operation. I was ready to move on. That wasn't too difficult for me to do. I have always tended to be forward-looking. I have always liked moving ahead to newer and bigger challenges; and what could be newer and bigger than high school?

You read about it in books. They make plays and movies about it. A lot of people say that high school was the best time of their life. A fresh start in a new building. New teachers and maybe some new friends. New girls. I could definitely look forward to that.

I was ready for high school.

Chapter Twenty: High School

I was 14 years old and ready for a fresh start. Since I was about to begin my first day in high school, I knew exactly what that meant. That meant that I was a freshman, a newbie, the bottom of the barrel. Need I say more? A lot of people warned me about that, and I always told them the same thing.

"If you think I don't know what it's like to be at the bottom of the barrel, guess again."

It didn't faze me one bit.

Hardly one week had passed into the semester when I began to grow restless. Classes occupied my time, but not enough of it. I needed something more to do. A lot of my friends were dating now, and I wasn't. Whenever I saw a couple, I thought back to the days when I was with Becca, and that made me restless. While I felt that I was finally used to the fact that we would never be together again, I wasn't ready to start a relationship with anyone else yet. So a little bit of extra activity would serve as a nice diversion for me.

I started exploring all the possibilities of what school had to offer a boy with too much energy. Since I could not play sports, my options were severely limited. I checked out the chess club, but that only lasted about a week. Something about chess did not excite me as much as I needed to be excited. There wasn't enough activity. I simply could not expend what was pent up inside me, so I had to move on. I kept searching and wishing for more excitement to enter my life. And, as the cliché goes, be careful for what you wish for. Fate decided to step in and force me to use up a lot of that energy.

It was a morning just like any other boring, old morning in the life of someone looking for a change. We were all in my van as Grandpa was making his usual rounds of delivering his grandkids to school. First, he would drop me at the high school, and then shoot on down the road to the junior high to drop off Cralynne. I was moaning and complaining about how dreary school had become, while Cray just sat there in the front seat, looking back at me and giggling, making a face once in a while just to see if she could make me laugh. It usually worked but not today.

Along the way, Grandpa noticed someone tailgating us, so he slowed down to be careful, as he was always someone who prided in taking care of his family. Grandpa has always taken his responsibilities very seriously. We pulled up right in front of the school, as usual, and we began the tedious and sometimes complicated process of exiting the van.

The rear door opened and the lift began sliding out so that I could back out onto it. My nurse was busy gathering my things, and Cralynne made one last attempt to cheer me up.

"Hey, C.V., don't beat anybody up," she said.

"Very funny," I replied.

"Don't kiss all the girls," she tried this time.

I didn't dignify that with a response, even though the thought of spending a day like that sounded like quite an improvement from

164

my current life.

"Anyhow, I hope you have a great day!" she added.

"Thanks," I mumbled under my breath, half-sarcastically.

The ramp in the van was unfolded and ready for me to get on it. My nurse was getting out of the van at this time, and Cralynne was in the front seat watching me, smiling as I prepared to make my exit.

The driver behind us was still causing problems for Grandpa and making things dangerous. He kept moving closer and closer to the van, and Grandpa kept watching him closely to make sure things were safe for me to exit. Grandpa then told me to back out, but he was not aware that he had already lowered the lift while he was watching the driver.

The lift was down only about 4 inches, but that was enough to cause a catastrophe. I began to back out, and when I did, my wheelchair flew straight backwards and down! In a split second of noise and movement and confusion, I was plunged into chaos. I dropped onto my back which sent the wheelchair sprawling backwards onto the lift with a harsh metal sound. This was accompanied by the screams of everyone who was watching; loudest of all was Cralynne's.

The weight and pressure of my heavy wheelchair caused the lift to drop straight to the ground. This caused my head to smack hard against the chair, which was "cushioned" by the metal of the lift and the concrete below. The rest of my body followed the momentum of the chair and headed in the general direction of my vulnerable head. My right leg flew off its leg rest, smashed hard into the side of the metal lift, and then caromed back into place on my wheelchair. The rest of my body absorbed the shock from the impact of the fall and then came to rest in the chair, which was now lying backwards upon the ground.

I had no idea what had happened. I was in a daze. My nurse was the first one to my side. She frantically tried to see what she could do. There was a huge commotion of sound all around me, as I lay still and tried to get my bearings.

"Are you okay?" she cried, "C.V., are you okay?"

"Oh, my God! C.V.! Oh, my God!" Grandpa screamed. "He's hurt! He's hurt!"

I could hear other sounds, people talking about what they saw and asking what happened. At that point, I began to feel like I was going to pass out. My eyes fluttered helplessly. Only the sounds of Cralynne crying snapped me out of it. Suddenly I was worried about her.

She saw the whole thing! I thought. *She saw me fall. Cralynne! Somebody help her!*

I was in tremendous pain and woozy, but all I could think about was my baby sister. That and how I felt like taking a short nap.

"Hey, C.V." yelled my nurse. "Don't you shut those eyes. You stay with me, mister. You stay with me! Do you hear me? Don't shut those eyes. You stay with me!"

I looked up at her and tried to say, "OK."

People kept running to and fro, encircling me with activity. Before I knew it, the school nurse were there, too. She started checking me out to assess the damage. They kept me completely still, being careful not to move me an inch just in case there was spinal cord damage. Then I heard the familiar sound of the ambulance.

During the commotion someone phoned 911, and the

emergency workers were there in no time. They asked about what had happened. I felt like saying "I tried to fly," in order to diffuse the situation and let them know that I was fine, but words couldn't come out. I wasn't fine.

The emergency workers looked me over and then made a quick decision. I had to get to a hospital right away. They lifted me off my wheelchair and placed me onto a stretcher, which was then gingerly placed into the ambulance.

No school today, I thought. *What a way to get out of it.*

The ambulance sped off with me inside and the workers trying to keep me from passing out. They tried to get me to speak but all I could think about was Cralynne...that and the pain.

My knee! My knee! Somebody fix my knee! I thought. *Cralynne? Where's Cralynne? If I die now, she'll be scarred forever. Cralynne! My knee. The pain!*

A few minutes later, we arrived at the Emergency Room and I was rushed directly in to be examined. Mom was already there, which puzzled me. I had no idea about how much time had elapsed. I still felt confused. All I knew was that everyone looked worried and very, very serious.

I'm going to die. I just know it, I thought. *How ironic. I survive a billion trips to the hospital. I survive pneumonia six times a year every year of my life. I survive the worst surgery ever. I survive all of that and then what kills me? I fall out of my van. If it didn't hurt so much, I would laugh.*

I had to stay on the backboard, strapped in tightly until they made sure my neck and back were stabilized. After a few minutes of examining me, the ER doctors had worried looks on their faces and I was sure that my biggest fear was about to come true. Then, one doctor informed my mom that he was concerned because when they

167

asked me to move my toes, I couldn't move them very much.

All of a sudden, Mom began to laugh out loud. That's when I started to feel better. If Mom was laughing, then there was no way that I was going to die.

The doctors looked at her like she was nuts. Then she explained to them about my disease, how people with SMA Type 1 would never be able to move their toes very much. The doctors looked relieved to hear that the accident hadn't caused me paralysis, but were still concerned about my overall condition. They felt that I should probably be transported by ambulance to University Hospital in Syracuse in order to receive more specialized care.

So, once again I was in my familiar mode of transportation, only this time there were no sirens and Mom was riding alongside me. This made it a little better, although I was still tightly strapped to the rock-hard backboard, feeling incredible pain in my knee, and wondering when the whole ordeal would be over. When we arrived in Syracuse, we went right into the Emergency Room. I began to tell them how much pain my knee was causing, and they told me my knee was fine and that they were concerned about my back. That's when I started to get impatient and annoyed.

I obviously had all my senses back, because the pain seemed to be getting worse and worse, and I was starting to clearly put into place the events of the day. Then, I thought of my sister.

"Where's Cralynne, Mom?" I asked.

"She's home with Grandpa," she answered. "She'll be fine."

"But she saw the whole thing. She was crying and…"

"She'll be fine. Grandpa will take good care of her."

I knew Mom was right. Grandpa took good care of everyone. And then it dawned on me: What if people blamed Grandpa?

"What about Grandpa?" I asked.

"What about him?"

"What if people blame him?"

"No one is going to blame Grandpa," Mom said. "It wasn't his fault. And even if they don't have the facts, everyone who knows him would know how well he takes care of you."

"I know, but some people might…"

"Since when did we start listening to some people?" Mom explained. "Don't worry about it. Let's just get you fixed up first."

I knew that the doctors would be concerned about my back, because it was only about a year earlier that I had the rod put in. I knew that they would focus on that. But my back felt fine to me. I knew that they would have to make sure and that was fine with me, as long as they paid attention to my knee – and as soon as possible. I tried telling them that my back was fine and it was my knee that hurt, but no one seemed to listen. In the meantime, the pain got worse and worse.

After close to six hours of lying there in excruciating pain, I finally got a break. The doctors came in and told me that there was no damage to my back. They told me that it was now time to check out my knee. I was so relieved when they at last wheeled me off to get it x-rayed. I was absolutely sure that something was wrong.

I was right. Sure enough a few minutes later, I got the news.

"Hello, Craig. How are you doing?" a doctor asked me.

169

I felt like saying, "How does it look like I am doing?" but I didn't. I just kept my mouth shut because I wanted some answers and I wanted them fast.

"Well, Craig, it looks like you're right," he said. "The reason your knee hurts is because it is broken."

At that point I felt like saying, "Duh!" but I didn't. At that point, I was beyond annoyed. I just wanted to get it fixed and have the pain stop. I just wanted to get out of there and go home. I just wanted an end to all the excitement. And I knew that it would be a long time before I wished for some again.

I was again carted off, this time to someplace called "the casting room." And since I hadn't seen any Hollywood producers or directors around, I figured that it was to get my knee fixed, and not to audition for a role in an upcoming feature film. Again I was right. Soon, I was face-to-face with a guy who was chock-full of bad jokes and plaster.

"Hey, there he is! There's the lucky boy!" he said, way too loudly to be taken seriously.

Lucky? I thought. *I'd hate to see the unlucky boy. Where was he, in the morgue? Anyhow, if this kind of luck continues, you'll never see me going to Las Vegas.*

I politely grinned and let him continue.

"Okay, let me see. Are you here for casting or for amputation?"

That one didn't deserve a laugh.

"One leg or two? Right or left or both?"

"Right," I said, just to get it over with.

170

"Okay, young man, let's patch you up. Now just don't run off on me while I'm working."

That was the worst yet. I didn't say another word until he was done.

So, after 10 hours – after being launched backwards into the air, two ambulance trips, seeing the insides of two Emergency Rooms, being examined by a hundred doctors, having a thousand x-rays, and listening to a million bad jokes – I was finally allowed to go home; bruised back, dented wheelchair, broken leg, and all.

On the ride home, I began to wonder how I would have to adjust to this hardship. It's tough enough being wheelchair-bound, simply because you have to rely on others to do everything for you. I'm the type of guy who would do things for myself if I could. At least my wheelchair was comfortable. The cast on my right knee was not.

Oh, well, I thought, *just another challenge. I will deal with it like I deal with everything else: Head on.*

I didn't really know what "head on" meant, but I knew that I would figure that out. I also knew that I wouldn't wish for more excitement in my life without qualifying that wish. From now on, any wishes for excitement would have to be without any doctors and loaded with pretty girls.

Oh yeah, I had it all figured out.

Chapter Twenty-One: Bros

I soon returned to school - wheelchair, cast, and all – and was looking for some brand new excitement that didn't involve a trip to the Emergency Room. At least that was the plan.

One of my teachers suggested that I check into the possibility of working at the school store. The school store was a place where students stopped by to purchase school supplies, chips, treats, fruit-flavored sugary-sweet snacks, and chocolate munchables – just the kinds of things that offered serious students a non-stop sugar rush to keep them going through the arduous school day. It was also a place where kids stopped by to hang out, waste time, or flirt with members of the opposite sex. It was my kind of place.

At first, I didn't think I had a shot at landing a job there. What real kind of work could I do? What did I have to offer? But I had a connection. One of the managers of the school store happened to be my homeroom teacher, so I decided to ask him if I had any chance of working there. I wasn't sure what kind of a reaction I would receive, but I am happy to say that it was positive. We talked for a while – a chat that was something close to an interview, but probably more of a formality than anything else – and then he offered me the job. He then took a look at my class schedule and penciled me in for work three times every week, at hours when he thought I could afford to be there. I was thrilled, eager to get to work, and even more eager to meet new people and have new adventures.

My first day at the store turned out to be one of the best days of my life. When I arrived, I realized that I didn't know a single person there. That was exactly what I wanted. One of the managers showed me around, basically told me to do whatever I could do, and that it really didn't matter much, as long as the work got done and no one got into trouble. That sounded pretty much like a license to goof off, or something close to it. It certainly sounded like all the rumors about the school store were true.

The first greetings I received from my fellow workers were polite, but chilly. Maybe they thought that I might be infringing upon their turf. It was also obvious that they were wondering what in the world I could ever do in the way of work. I can understand why they would think that way.

It didn't take long before things began to get friendlier.

"Hey," a guy said, matter-of-factly, as he ran his hand along the arm of my chair.

"Hey," I answered, not knowing if I was about to be confronted.

"What're you in for?" he asked.

"In for?"

"Yeah, Bro, how'd you get the job?"

"Oh. My homeroom teacher is one of the managers," I

explained.

"Cool," he said, nodding his approval and looking me over.

"Yeah, cool."

His name was J.T. and he was (and still is) one of the coolest people I have ever met in my entire life. In fact, though we don't look much alike at all, when I look at J.T., I see myself, or the kind of person that I would be if I could walk and didn't have adults with me all the time. Deep inside, I felt like he could be my twin. The two of us hit it off immediately.

J.T. was two years older than me, but only one year ahead of me in school. He was on the tall side and very muscular, with deep, dark, wavy black hair. He was the kind of guy at whom the girls always stared when he walked by. That alone impressed me. But there were so many other things that I found intriguing about him. J.T. had his ears pierced in three places, a tongue ring, and four tattoos. Need I say more? J.T. fascinated me right from the start.

"So, how long you been in the chair?" he asked.

"Almost all my life."

"Cool. Any chance of getting out?"

"No, not really. According to the doctors, I should've been dead a long time ago."

"Cool," he continued. "My kind of guy. A survivor."

"Yeah, I guess," I said. "I guess you could describe me that way."

"So, how much can you move?" he asked straight out.

"Not too much. My feet hardly at all. My head barely. Only

my forearms and hands a little," I explained.

"Not a problem. So, then what do you do?"

"Well, I basically just try stuff out and see what I can and can't do. I'll try almost anything. Sometimes we invent new ways of doing things. I like to take chances. If it works, it works. If it doesn't, it doesn't. That's about it."

"Cool."

"Yeah."

"Oh, by the way, the name's J.T. You?"

"C.V."

Right then and there I saw we had a lot in common besides initials: the honesty, the direct way of speaking, and the lack of fear. Then a girl walked past and he quickly took his focus off of me, staring at her all the way down the hall. That's when I knew that we had more than a lot in common.

Since we were to be working together at exactly the same times every week, it didn't take very long for the two of us to get to know one another and to become close friends. That friendship spilled over to classes that we had together, time spent in and out of class, and then time spent out of school. J.T. would come over to my house all the time; and we spent hour after hour hanging out.

We both had a great love for music; talking about it and listening to it took up a good portion of our time, only surpassed by the time we spent talking about girls, our number one favorite thing to do next to actually *being* with girls. We were both huge fans of heavy metal, only J.T. dressed the part a little better than I did, unless of course you want to count my wheelchair as part of the outfit. That was some pretty heavy metal. Many an afternoon was spent listening to the latest releases and giving them a "thumbs up" or a "thumbs down." And, to be completely honest, we sometimes used the same system when we were talking about girls.

The only thing J.T. and I ever had a mild disagreement about also happened to be related to music. You see, J.T. had a fondness for country music, which never quite appealed to me. Try as he might to get me to like it, he never succeeded. As far as I was concerned, it was Metallica or it was nothing. Heavy metal was what I loved.

Of course, we didn't just talk about music or girls – though, really, what else was there? But once in a while we would have conversations about life, about how difficult it can be at times. It was easy to open up to J.T., as he felt closer to me than a brother. It was more like looking in the mirror or having a talk with your conscience. Both of us could say anything that we wanted and we knew that not a single word would ever leave the room. We respected each other that much.

One day, J.T. admitted to me that he was a recovering drug user. I didn't quite know how to react when he told me that. I knew it was probably hard to say, so I just sat there and listened to his story. He told me all about his struggles and how he had made the decision to get clean. I admired him for his honesty, and I admired him because I knew he had accomplished what he set out to do. J.T. didn't do drugs anymore.

One of J.T.'s favorite things to do was to flirt. Who am I kidding? It was everyone's favorite thing to do. The only difference is that J.T. had a distinct flair for it. As soon as he saw a cute girl in line, he would go into his act. He would get a different sort of look on his face, and I always knew what that meant: girl alert! I actually think he got taller when a girl was around. At least that is how it looked from my vantage point.

And if it meant having a few extra seconds to look at a girl, boy would J.T. slow down to a crawl. He'd slowly walk to the shelves and pretend that he couldn't find whatever it was she wanted to buy, even though everyone could tell that he never once took his eyes off of her. And of course, he would then drop the money on the floor, only if to look over at me and give me a wink and a sly smile. Yes, J.T. had a thing for the ladies.

Getting to know the people at the school store was such a pleasure, but getting to know everyone else wasn't. J.T. liked to introduce me around. It was his way of showing me the ropes and how to handle high school. It was his way of protecting me. And in a real sense, J.T. became what one might consider to be my bodyguard.

I never had any real problems with people unless they were phony or had an agenda. I didn't have the patience for that. If someone wanted to give me a hard time for any reason, well I would just as soon not waste my time with them. Life was too precious to waste on idiots. And high school, like the real world, had its fair share of idiots.

If I had to generalize and apply labels, I would say that there were three groups of people with whom I didn't get along very well: the jocks, the preppies, and the bullies. Bullies have bothered me from as far back as I can remember, and I think they always will. I cannot stand for that type of behavior at all. Preppies always seemed shallow to me. Anyone whose life focus was on wearing the right clothes, the latest hairstyle, or designer sunglasses wasn't worth wasting my breath on. I ignored them and they ignored me.

I had a problem with a few jocks that ignoring simply could not solve. Realistically, there wasn't much I had in common with someone involved in sports. Oh, I do enjoy watching sports on television, know enough about athletics to hold my own in a conversation, and have always had a secret desire to know what it

178

would feel like to play hockey; but other than that, I'm not jock material. I didn't hang out with them and they didn't hang out with me.

Jocks appeared to rule my high school. They got most of the attention as well as the cute girls. From time to time, there would be trouble between me and a jock. I think that was out of jealousy. Some jocks (and others, too) just did not like the attention that came my way because of my illness and my chair. In some ways, I threatened them. It is quite possible that their ego was so fragile that it became deflated easily. In their quest for attention by focusing on achieving the perfect body, they could not handle the fact that someone who did not have one was also getting attention.

One day, that jealousy sprouted into confrontation. It all took place between classes, the time when all the cliques of the school entangled head-on in a mad dash of energy and chaos. Things are bound to unravel when you have all of that happening in close quarters, especially in a high school hallway. And it did.

A kid who did not like me from day one of my high school life, a jock with a perpetually bad attitude, stumbled upon me as I made my way to class. On that particular day, he decided that he had the need to get in my face and take me down a few notches. Who knows why he decided to confront me at precisely that moment? Maybe he was having a bad day and needed his ego boosted. Maybe his girlfriend broke up with him in favor of an even more muscular Neanderthal. Or maybe he forgot to have his hourly dose of raw meat. No matter what, he charged me in a split second.

I don't recall the exact exchange of insults; but I am sure that I held my own. Verbally, I can be pretty fierce in defending myself if the need arises. Oh, I am certain that he made a few clever remarks about me being handicapped or having physical limitations. And I am quite sure that he hadn't realized that I had heard it all before, and

179

that I did not let the remarks of idiots bother me. I volleyed back with a few remarks about being muscle-bound between the ears and such things. But I wasn't certain that he understood the meaning of my words. I quickly realized that I had to lower my vocabulary to his level to get my point across.

I called him a jerk. That he understood. He called me a cripple. I sidestepped it with ease. I called him stupid, and he proved my point.

"Oh yeah? Oh yeah?" he scowled at me. "You think you're so smart with your nurse and your chair and all your friends. You'll see! You'll see!"

"What are *you* gonna do to *me?*" I quipped sarcastically. He thought for a second – for a long second. He was confused.

"I'll tell you what I'm gonna do. I'll pop those tires and let all the air out. Yeah. I'll slash 'em. How d'you like that, you cripple? Huh?" he smiled.

All I could do was to laugh. In fact I began to howl. This made him even angrier.

"You idiot," I said loud enough for everyone in the hallway to hear, "There's no air in these tires. They're filled with foam. You can't pop them. It's impossible. What an idiot!"

By that time a large crowd was laughing at him, only making him fume. He came even closer and, at that point, I actually thought he was going to do me some physical harm.

"Well then, maybe I will just have to pop you," he threatened. "Don't think I won't. I'll hit a cripple."

"You'll hit a cripple?!" said a voice in the crowd. "You'll hit a cripple!"

It was J.T., who had just arrived in time to hear the last few threatening words. He wasted no time at all in jumping into the fray. He didn't ask for an explanation. He didn't feel the need to sort things out. He felt the need to protect me.

J.T. grabbed the guy by the shoulders and hurled him across the hall toward the lockers. He pinned him there by his throat and began lifting him up. By that time, my muscular foe was scared, to put it mildly.

"If you ever lay one hand on him…"

J.T. paused for a second or two. You could feel the anger seething in him. It was so palpable you could almost taste it.

"If you ever lay one hand on him…"

Again he paused. I don't think there were words strong enough to convey the intensity of what he was feeling at that moment. It didn't matter. He had everyone shaking in their shoes. I began checking under my jock friend for a puddle.

"If you ever lay one hand on him…you're dead."

I am one hundred percent certain that J.T. did not mean that he would kill the guy. He just picked those words because nothing much trumps them. I do, however, believe that he would have beaten up the guy pretty thoroughly. There was no doubt about that. And, come to think of it, the words he chose didn't matter that much. The jock got the message, his jock friends got the message, and so did everyone who witnessed the scene. After that, I was left alone for quite some time. As far as the jerks at the school were concerned, anywhere near me was a "bully-free zone."

181

The rest of my freshman year was uneventful. That was fine by me. One trip to the Emergency Room and one death threat per semester was enough excitement to last me a while. I began to get even more excited about my music, if that was possible. I was in chorus again, and to my delight, J.T. had joined as well. We could have been clones. We did everything together. Life with J.T. and all my new friends was a dream come true. Life at the school store was just too much fun to be imagined. I cherished these days of pure fun and happiness. I wanted them to go on forever.

Chapter Twenty-Two: Alex

The euphoria of my freshman year did not carry over into my sophomore year. Something was missing in my life. I was bored with school. I was restless, distracted and lost with no clue why. I started acting out, rebelling. I was a loose cannon, and my disease only made it worse. That's because when some people see a person in a wheelchair, they let them get away with murder.

My grades began to slip. I fell behind in my homework. One teacher had noticed this and stepped in right away. She grounded me from going to the school store for two weeks. Two weeks of no J.T. Two weeks of no friends. You would have thought that I would have gotten the message by that point, but you would have been wrong.

More and more I had this feeling of frustration inside me. More and more I began acting out. And it seemed like my bodyguard, J.T., was right there beside me every time. Most of the time it was minor stuff, nothing at all like getting into fights or causing damage. Why, we hardly ever got into trouble. But a few times, we were not what you would call "model students."

I guess that both of us have always had a problem in putting up with other people's "garbage." I wouldn't call it a matter of the two of us being impatient or even rebellious. It was just that when people treated us a certain way, or if we felt wronged or even mistreated, we didn't stand for it. And that meant that sometimes we would talk too much in class...or worse.

A few times, late in the school day, we cut school. I would make up some excuse like I had to go to the bathroom, or that I had to go someplace to get something, and then we would both pick up and leave the school. I know that it was wrong to do. I know that we both should have been punished. But no one ever did. No one ever had the guts to punish us. And that is what I mean by saying I was mistreated.

When you think of being mistreated, you usually think of some kind of mean or evil thing happening to a person. But it isn't always like that. Sometimes when you do something wrong and people look the other way, that is also a form of mistreatment. It is nothing more than people not treating you the same way as everyone else. That is something that has always bothered me. I wanted to be treated just like everyone else. So, skipping out of classes was just my dumb way of saying, "If you are going to treat me differently, then I'll take advantage of it and see how you like it." It was my way of testing people and pushing the limits.

And I liked to push the limits.

Sophomore year ended like that, a little rebellious, a little confused. Little did I realize that my restlessness wasn't from boredom at school. It was a result of what was lacking in my life. And what was lacking was a relationship with a girl.

The month of June was dwindling down to its last few days, causing students to grow itchy with anticipation of that last dismissal bell. I was looking forward to a lazy summer of sleeping late, listening

184

to tunes, and turning sixteen – nothing much else – when I got invited to attend the junior high school graduation of my sister Cralynne and my cousin David, one of my closest buddies in the whole world. It was a proud day for my family, and I was excited to go, so I eagerly said "yes."

That day changed my life forever.

During the ceremony, my wandering eye spotted this beautiful girl amidst the several hundred who were about to graduate. Stunningly blonde, she was easily the most beautiful girl I had ever seen in my entire life. Try as I might, I could not manage to pay attention to the ceremony. I could not take my eyes off her. Every so often, I would glance at the podium, or feign paying attention to the proceedings, but it was no use. She had captivated me. I watched as she spoke to the girl next to her and they shared a laugh. I watched her as she touched her finger to her cheek. I followed her as she walked to the stage and received her diploma. I could not do anything else but give my full attention to this beauty. It was like watching an angel who'd come down to earth.

The ceremony ended much too soon, leaving me with the uneasy feeling that I would never see a vision such as her again. Sure enough, as the crowd started to disperse, and everyone made their way to the exits, I lost her. I felt saddened, but I told myself that such things were inevitable. I would always have her in my fantasies, for as long as they lasted.

After graduation, people were milling about in the parking lot, congratulating each other and saying their summer farewells; while I sat, waiting hopefully that I would get another chance to see her. As luck would have it, she walked in my direction, approaching me along with her mother. The two of them gazed straight at me and smiled as they walked by.

I wanted to speak up. I wanted to shout out. Something. Anything. But I didn't. I couldn't. What could I say that would not sound foolish?

"Hey, you. You're beautiful." Or perhaps, *"I could fall for someone like you."*

No. No way. They sounded too much like pickup lines. And I didn't feel like saying anything that didn't sound dead serious.

I sat there, dumbfounded and awkward, itching with every fiber of my being to speak up. Yet I didn't. All that I could manage was a friendly smile back as they passed by, found their car and disappeared forever. All that I was left with was her smile.

About a week later there was a knock on my bedroom door. My bedroom was near the back of the house on the left side, recessed a little from the street. It had its own door that led outside, which made it great for having friends over without bothering anyone else in the house (and also great if someone wanted to sneak in to see me without having my family notice).

My cousin Dave was at the door. Dave and I have always been close. We are more like brothers than cousins, since neither one of us has a biological brother. We hang out all the time, playing video games against each other, and listening to music. We also share thoughts and feelings about our lives that we have sworn never to tell anyone. So I won't start by blabbing now.

At first I thought Dave had stopped by to see if he could whip me at my latest video game, but that wasn't the reason. He had a request, one that seemed very strange at the time. You see, Dave had been interested in a particular girl in his class for a long time. He told me that her name was Alex, short for Alexandra, and that she was gorgeous. He admitted that he had spoken to her several times and that he wasn't making any progress in getting her to go out with him. So, he essentially wanted me to be his "wing man." He wanted me to call her up and say a million great things about him to see if I could get her interested in him.

My first reaction was that it was a lame idea and it would never work. But stranger things have happened, so I agreed to do it. I knew that people said I had a way with words, so I figured that if I laid it on thick and said what a great guy he was, I might be able to help him out. I would do almost anything to help him out. Plus I felt that I didn't have to lie, because I already thought he was a great guy.

I agreed to do it, thinking that in the long run it could help both of us out. What if Alex knew that girl I had seen at graduation? What if I was lucky enough that they were friends? Maybe she could give me her phone number, or put in a good word about me. It was worth a shot. Visions of us double-dating started running through my head. What if we both found the girls of our dreams? How awesome that would be! I was on the phone in no time.

I will admit I was a tiny bit nervous about calling Alex up to talk about Dave. What would I say to break the ice? How could I avoid appearing awkward or foolish?

My fears were unfounded. Dave had certainly chosen someone who was easy to talk to. I just introduced myself as Dave's cousin and asked her if we could talk a bit. Alex agreed. Minutes seemed to fly by like seconds. We chatted briefly before I started directing the conversation toward the goal: Dave. She didn't seem to be interested at that point, so I didn't push the issue. I asked if it would be alright to call back at another time and she agreed.

The next time I called, I knew I had to do a better job of "selling" Dave to her. Again, we talked for a while. The conversation was relaxed and easy, and could have gone on all day. Alex's voice was warm and enticing. It made me wonder what she looked like. It made me wonder if her face was as beautiful as she sounded on the phone.

But, the devoted cousin that I am, I again directed the conversation to the topic of Dave. Alex quickly cooled down. Then I said straight out the reason that I had called her in the first place. Alex did not act shocked or annoyed, but she did make it clear that she was not interested in my cousin, and had no desire in him for the future. She was not going to go out with him. That was that.

It was time to tell Dave the bad news. I worried about how hard he would take it. I knew that he had tried for a long time to talk to Alex. I knew how much he wanted to get her to go out with him and I didn't want to hurt his feelings. Sure enough, when I told Dave the news, he was crushed. But things were about to get worse.

I tried to make him feel better about losing Alex, but that was difficult to do. From my phone conversations with her, I could already tell how wonderful a person she was. I had enjoyed those conversations so much; though I knew mentioning that to Dave would only make matters worse. We talked for a while; and I used every cliché in the book. I talked about moving on, all the fish in the sea, and about putting your eggs in one basket; though I think I got a couple of the clichés wrong. Dave got the message: Alex was not going to go out with him, and it was better to move on.

Still, I could not help but wonder what Alex looked like, so I admitted to Dave how nice the chats had been, and that I was curious to see if her face matched her voice. He told me that he would show me a picture if I wanted. I agreed and we both figured that would put an end to the whole thing.

The next day, Dave came over with his yearbook. My heart skipped a beat, thinking that I would finally get a glimpse of Dave's not-so-secret crush. He thumbed through the pages until he found her picture. Then he put the book in front of me and pointed her out. And my heart skipped a thousand beats.

It was her! It was the girl from graduation, the one that I could not take my eyes off. Alex was that girl! What was I to do now? I had talked to her. I knew that I wanted her, but how could I tell Dave without losing him forever? How do I tell him that I was interested in the same girl that he was, without making it seem that I had stabbed him in the back? How could I break his heart twice?

I thought about it for a while, and then figured that the best thing to do would be to behave the same way I would with anything: tackle it head on, speak the plain truth, and get it out in the open as quickly as possible. Then, if problems arose, we would deal with them. This is the way to face life. So, with some apprehension, I told Dave that I wanted to date Alex.

I told him that she was the girl I had seen at graduation, the same beauty that I had told him about right after it happened. Dave knew that I wasn't just making this up in order to get my chance with her. Dave knew all along about that girl because I never stopped talking about her.

To say that Dave was not pleased would be like calling a monsoon a passing shower. He was beyond upset. It was one thing to have a girl say "no" to you, but another thing – another way worse thing – to have her say "yes" to one of your best friends. No matter what happened, the road ahead was going to be bumpy for a while.

We spent a lot of hours – just the two of us – talking this out. We didn't hold back. Eventually, Dave calmed down and said that he would not be angry if I asked Alex out. I could tell that he still had pain in his heart as he told me. He was being a good sport about it. He even wished me good luck. Dave had realized that Alex could just as easily turn me down, too, something that never crossed my mind at all. As soon as the air was cleared, I called Alex and we picked up right where we left off, laughing, joking, and talking about school. Only this time the conversation was not headed toward asking her to go out with my cousin, it was headed toward asking her to go out with me.

It's hard to describe what was going through my head at that time. My emotions were running on overdrive. I am not one to talk about such things as "love at first sight," and I would never say that I fell in love with Alex when I saw her back at graduation. But I do know that something magical happened to me that day. It was like being struck in the heart by lightning and your whole perspective on life changes. It's like looking out of the window on rainy days and all you can see is the sun. You feel things that you never knew existed and that's what I felt when I first saw Alex. And, though I didn't know what my chances with her would be, I knew that nothing was going to stop me from trying to get closer to her.

I continued calling Alex on a regular basis. And, even though we hit it off immediately, there were hurdles in my path. Alex admitted that she had two other boys interested in her. They were both in her class, and had been paying her quite a bit of attention for some time. At that point, she hadn't made up her mind which boy she wanted to date, but at least I was included in the top three.

So, it was a competition against two freshmen for the most beautiful woman on the planet. I don't like competition. Well, that's not exactly true, I don't mind competitions, losing I couldn't stand! I made up my mind, right then and there, to try even harder to win her affection. And I would do it the best way that I knew how: by being myself.

I found out that Alex lived only about half a mile from my house and I kept thinking about how easy it would be to go from house to house, how easy it would be to see each other whenever we wanted. But she hadn't said "yes" yet. I had to be patient.

I also had my pal J.T. in my corner to help me. He coached me about the "ins and outs" of getting a girl to like you. With an older guy coaching me, those poor freshmen didn't stand a chance. After talking for a few days more, we noticed that we were both very interested in each other. I could feel her start to sway. It was just a matter of time. And after some time, it happened. I'll never forget the moment. It meant so much to me that I had the presence of mind to look at the clock, making a mental note of the exact date and time that she said "yes." It was Wednesday night, June 29th, 2005, at 10:06 p.m. That was the moment that Alex told me told me that she wanted to date me. I was the happiest that I had been in a very long time.

Now that Alex had agreed to date me, it was time to schedule a date. We decided that she would come over to my place the following Friday. Oh how I wished I could skip the next few days! I know I should be more patient, but life is short and why wait to do what you want?

Alex and her mom arrived at my house around noon on that Friday. The first thing that I noticed when she entered our living room was that she was even more beautiful than I had remembered. I can clearly recall what she was wearing: pink Capri pants and a pink and white tank top – because I never took my eyes off her for a second. She stood about 5 foot 5 and was very thin. I doubt if she even weighed 100 pounds. Her blonde hair hung down past her shoulders and framed her face perfectly, complimenting the most sparkling pair of blue eyes that I had ever seen. In fact, all of her sparkled. She had an air that was unbelievably captivating, more beautiful than a movie star. She had the kind of looks that have inspired artists to paint paintings, photographers to take pictures, and

191

men who do not have such beauty in their lives to go crazy. I doubt that any male could ever resist her. I knew that, if we were to ever become serious, I would have my work cut out for me.

The first few minutes were polite, but awkward. They were filled with the pleasantries of families getting to know one another. Alex's mom introduced herself to my grandparents, and everyone just sat there for a while, chatting. Alex and I sat quietly, exchanging glances, both secretly wondering if we would ever get any time together alone. Finally after a while, her mom left and I brought her back into my living area.

We were both shy at first, but eventually we both began to open up.

"So, this is where you live," Alex observed.

"Yeah, they built onto the house when I started getting too big to be taken care of in the main section. My chair moves around better in my living area," I explained.

"Cool. And that's your TV, and that's your bed."

"Yeah, that's where I sleep," I answered, thinking that the conversation wasn't making much progress. "I really like your outfit," I continued.

"Thanks. You don't think it's too pink do you?"

"No, I love it."

"Do you like pink?"

"On girls I do."

She smiled. She got my joke. Things were going well.

As the day went on, the conversation became more and more

relaxed. It didn't take us long to get to the comfort point that we had reached during our telephone chats. In fact, we grew close to one another amazingly fast – "movie fast" – where you only have 90 minutes to cram in a whole lifetime. That's how it felt: rapid and smooth…and just perfect.

Alex and I had similar views about life and the world around us, but there were a few areas in which we did not see eye to eye: though we both loved music and were in chorus, she played an instrument – the violin – and I did not. And though we both loved listening to the latest songs, her tastes were a bit softer than mine. She liked country music, which I never had a taste for.

The talking continued, hour upon hour, and soon Alex was sitting close to me as we continued to get to know each other. Her mom had gone home, and the other adults respected us enough to allow us our privacy. This turned out to be a very good thing indeed, as in the early evening we shared our first kiss.

It was like something from a storybook, where, as soon as your lips touch, birds fly out from everywhere and take to the sky, flowers shower down from the heavens, and an orchestra starts playing in the background. That's how perfect a kiss it was. I could not help but wonder if our first kiss was that good, what would our second be like? And our third? And our fourth? I hoped that I would find out soon.

By the end of the evening we were cuddling and talking, though I will admit the cuddling began to dominate the talking both in amount and importance. It felt so good having Alex touch me. I never wanted it to end, but it did. Around 11 p.m. she went home and I was left with the feeling that I had already fallen in love. That was all it took for me: one perfect day. And I was left to dream about what the future would have in store for us.

Chapter Twenty-Three: Bliss

Bright and early the next morning, Alex's mom dropped her off at my house. She spent the entire day with me. And the next day. And the day after that. Soon we were inseparable and our lives intertwined. I learned everything about her and she learned everything about me; including all about my illness, my machines, and my daily regimen – not because she had to, but because she *wanted* to. Alex began doing many of the same tasks that my nurses usually did and she did them well, always smiling and cheerful.

Life became absolutely perfect, if that is at all possible. It was summer and we were young and in love. Soon Alex began coming over in the morning and sneaking quietly into my bed while I was still asleep. She would wrap her arms around me, cuddling closely as I slowly awoke. The first time that she did this, I thought I was either dreaming or I had died and gone to Heaven. It was like a thousand birthday presents all wrapped into one. Alex came dressed with a bow each and every day. She was God's gift to me.

I was like a child on Christmas morning. Once you start opening presents, you want to keep going and never stop. You become addicted to the non-stop bliss. You crave it each and every second that you breathe. I needed Alex's touch and could think of nothing else.

I remember how Alex would lean me forward in my wheelchair just to hug me. She would carefully loosen my straps and gently move my body toward hers. Then we would stay like that, holding each other for hours at a time. We both needed that closeness. We could not stand to be apart. But it went beyond the physical. It went beyond mere teenage love. It felt real. It felt permanent. Many an afternoon we would cuddle while watching a movie and Alex would whisper "I love you" in my ear. I had never felt anything so wonderful in my life. It was sheer bliss.

Soon my chair was becoming a hindrance to our relationship. It was a reality of my life that I had always dealt with, and dealt with positively. But in order for me to be even closer to Alex – something that I desperately wanted – I needed more and more time out of my chair. I am happy to say that this was something that both my family and most of my nurses completely understood. They knew what I needed and were not about to put any more roadblocks in my path. They didn't make me beg for the freedom that I needed. They allowed it to occur naturally and normally. They even made it easy.

"I need to stretch," I would say. And, while stretching was something that was part of my usual therapy and encouraged in order to keep me healthy and avoid further physical deterioration, that was not what I was asking for. To my caretakers, "I need to stretch" meant that I wanted to be out of my chair so that I could be physically closer to Alex. This meant unstrapping me from my chair and placing me someplace – the couch, a large comfy chair, my bed – and making me comfortable so that Alex could hold me and we could be intimate.

"I need to stretch" was not the only signal that I used to tell people what was on my mind. When I felt certain urges, I would sing a Christmas carol or two, which had special meanings that everyone knew. This was my way of saying that I needed some private time with Alex so that we could be intimate. Everyone understood and allowed this. All it took was a few bars of "Jingle Bells" and the room would clear.

During those times, my nurse would leave and allow us to have our privacy as long as we wanted. The only stipulation was that she would need to be close enough to hear me if I had to call for help. Other than that, we were all alone: Alex, me, and our young love. And we did experience love. There was nothing that we did not do. Our physical love was as real as our emotional love.

More and more, Alex became my world. She was everything that I needed, everything that I could ever want. Alex wanted to satisfy all of my needs, which was fine by me, but occasionally someone would see it another way. The more familiar she would become with my machines, the more some nurses would speak up. It was not a case of jealousy. It was a case of them worrying about what could happen if I was left in the hands of someone with no medical training. A few nurses would watch Alex carefully as she tended to me. She never made a mistake. She was so meticulous that some became comfortable with having her do some things for me. Others were not. A few of my nurses left because of this, one had to be fired because she left the premises to do some errands, which was against regulations. But most stayed and adjusted to the situation.

A few months into our relationship, toward the unofficial end of the summer, the Great New York State Fair was set to take place. The Fair is always held in Syracuse because of its central location, and is a big occasion for us Central New Yorkers. It is a fun-filled mix of exhibits of all sorts, food, rides, and musical performances. During its ten days, it usually attracted hundreds of thousands of people from all over. Alex and I felt like this would be a good time for us to step out into the world – together.

One of the exhibits at the State Fair was the classic cars exhibit. And since both Alex's dad and Mark, my stepdad, had cars in the show, we wanted to attend. This was one of our first big public outings and it was very exciting. At first, I wasn't sure what people would think, not that I cared, not that it would stop me from being with the one that I loved. I was just curious to see the reaction, and curious to see how Alex would be in public. I wondered if she would treat me the same way that she did when we were alone and no one could see us. And I am glad to say that she did.

I remember us walking around the Fair, and how she did not hesitate to take my arm off of my arm rest and hold my hand in public. I was not expecting it. It made me so proud to know that she would treat me like this. I was so happy to see that she was not afraid to say "this is my man and I love him." That is what I loved about Alex: she was not afraid. She was so loving, caring, and giving, and not afraid to show it.

Regretfully, others were not of the same mind as Alex. There were plenty of stares that came in our direction, along with a fair share of smiles. Still, I would much rather have gone through the crowd unnoticed, unless the stares were from guys who were jealous that I could be with such a beauty. I could do without the smiles of pity, or the "aren't they cute" kind of smiles. The looks of bewilderment also annoyed me, as if they were saying "how could someone like you get a girl like her?"

Face it. I could and I did. Now accept me, be jealous of me, or get out of my way. My lady and I want to enjoy the Fair.

A few days later we were back visiting the Fair. My birthday had been about two weeks prior to that and my mom had gotten me tickets to see a concert at the grandstand. The group Nickelback was playing. I liked them a lot; but I liked the opening act, Crossfade, even more. They were one of my favorites. When I heard that they were playing at the Fair, I was hoping that someone would take me. And when I discovered that my Mom had gotten tickets for Alex, me, and my nurse, Debbie, who had been one of my caregivers most of my life, I was beside myself with happiness. I could hardly wait for the day to arrive. Music and my girl. What could be better than that?

The day of the concert came and we drove to Syracuse for the show. As soon as I was out of my van, I made a beeline straight for the gate, causing Alex and Debbie a bit of a hardship trying to keep up with me. I guess at that point, proper etiquette escaped me. A guy should never leave his girl behind like that, not even for the best band on earth…not even for Metallica.

The two caught up to me and shot a few nasty glances in my direction. I got the message right away. *Slow down. Okay I get it, but do you realize how hard it is to slow down?* I thought. I did slow down, but still kept a brisk pace as I weaved through the crowd.

Once inside the grandstand venue, we made our way to our seats, which, much to my delight, were in the front row! We were remarkably close to the speakers, something which thrilled me, but undoubtedly caused my companions for the evening to have cause for alarm, having somewhat "tamer" tastes in music than I did. I was looking forward to several hours of thunderous, metallic distortion, booming, fuzzed power chords, and ear-piercing leads. Alex and my nurse looked a bit less excited at the prospect of extended hearing loss.

"Wow, first row," Alex observed.

"Yeah. I am psyched," I replied.

"We're pretty close," she continued.

"Very close," my nurse added.

"Yeah, I know. This is awesome! I'm gonna have to thank Mom again. These are the best seats ever!"

"Yeah, very close," said Alex with a bit of trepidation.

"What, are you worried about something, baby?" I asked, smiling because I already knew what the problem was.

"No, not really."

"Good, 'cause there won't be any twangy voices or steel guitar tonight," I added with a sly smile. "Just head-banging metal."

"Um, yeah, good…I guess."

"Relax," I said, knowing that my teasing wasn't helping. "You'll love it. Just sit back and let the music take you away. Relax and fly."

Alex smiled at me. I knew that she would give it her best shot. She knew that if I loved heavy metal, it was important for her to try and love it, too (Fortunately, I never had to admit to her that I didn't feel the same need to try and love country music).

The night finally came upon us. It was show time. Colored lights came up and the band took the stage. As the first chord was struck and the sound waves from the speakers shook us to the core, Alex took my hand. I looked at her and smiled. Then she reached her head toward mine and whispered something soft in my ear. But since the band was about a thousand times louder than she was, I have no idea what she said. But, my heart has always known for sure it was to say that she loved me.

There was never a more perfect evening. The music was exquisite. The night air warm with just a hint of crispness as the hour grew late. Everyone was having a great time. I even managed to catch a guitar pick, which was tossed into the crowd for a souvenir, as it landed right on me. Once in a while, my nurse would wander off a few yards, just to give us a little "privacy," or as much privacy as anyone could have in a crowd of thousands of people. Still, we appreciated the gesture. Alex would hold my hand or run her fingers up and down my arm. I will admit that a few times she almost distracted me from the music…almost. I guess a woman can do that. A woman makes a music all her own, even louder and more powerful than when speakers are right in front of you.

Right around the time that the concert was ending and everyone had to leave, My nurse came to us with some exciting news. It seems that when she was giving us a moment alone, she had bumped into a member of Crossfade, who was walking around. He noticed my nurse from when she was sitting beside me, and asked about me. She told him how I was the group's biggest fan, and when he heard that, he invited us backstage to meet the band.

You can just about imagine how excited I was when I heard that. If I could have moved my legs, I would have sprung out of my chair and leapt for joy. Forget that, if I could have, I would have rocketed to the moon and back!

As soon as my nurse told me, I was off like a bolt of lightning. Then it dawned upon me that I didn't know where backstage was, so I had to wait for everyone else. We found our way backstage, met the band, and even had our picture taken with them. It was the best night of my life…to that point. It seemed like I had a habit of saying that every night that I was with Alex.

With the end of the New York State Fair came the end of summer and the start of yet another school year. Neither one of us was looking forward to that at all. In fact, we dreaded it. We were worried that school would dramatically cut back on the amount of time we could spend together, and we were right. Alex was a freshman and I was a junior. We wouldn't have any classes together and there was no way to do homework together if you were in different classes. Even Chorus could not bring us together because we were in different choruses, and we wouldn't be singing together. We didn't feel like going back. Instead, we felt like running away to our own private place and being together all the time. Just the two of us. Forever.

Amazingly, both of our families realized how important it was for our relationship to continue. They did everything they could to help us find time to be together. Alex was dropped off at my house in the mornings just so she could spend some time with me before school. We would then ride together in my van, splitting up only as we headed different ways during the day. We set up meeting times throughout the day just so we could be close for a few minutes. At the end of the day, she rode home with me and spent most of the day there. It was a start.

Then, more allowances were made. At the time, Alex and I did not realize how special they were and how privileged we were to receive them. The school provided us with a classroom just so we could have our lunch together and not make us eat in the cafeteria like everyone else. They allowed us to be alone. Now that I think back, I am almost embarrassed about it because we were receiving special treatment. But at the time, what did I care? All I knew is that it meant we could be together and that was all that mattered.

The two of us would sit there quietly in the empty classroom and enjoy our lunch. At least I think we enjoyed our lunch. When I look back, I cannot remember taking a single bite of food. All I can remember is Alex. My nurse would wander outside the classroom, giving us privacy, but staying within earshot. But all I needed during those times was to be alone with Alex. She and I would talk a bit; but mostly we got to be close. She would run her fingers through my hair or stroke my cheek. And sometimes – well lots of times – when no one was looking, she would kiss me. This is how school should be for everyone. If school was like this for every student, I don't know if anyone's grades would improve, but at least absenteeism would stop.

I supposed you could say that I was becoming selfish. We both were. All that we could think about was being together; and if that meant taking advantage of the generosity of others, we did it. If that meant neglecting a friend now and then, so be it. As far as we were concerned, we were the ones for each other. We talked about our future, getting married, having kids – everything. That is how serious we were about our relationship.

Our families both respected our relationship and the seriousness with which we approached it. In looking back, I often wonder if they just humored us, thinking that it was a phase we were going through. I often wonder why they never said a single word to slow us down or give us caution. After all, I was 16 and Alex was about to turn 15. It's hard to make life plans at such a tender age. But we wanted to try.

In retrospect, I wonder if Alex's family welcomed me with open arms because they saw my chair and thought that I was a "safe" boy for her to date, or was it true affection for me? I always thought that they were loving people with the best intentions. They have always treated me well and I quickly felt like I was around family when I was with them.

My first visit to Alex's house was the weekend before she turned 15. I loved being able to go to her house. It was like having our relationship affirmed; receiving the stamp of approval, and seeing it grow right before our eyes. It felt like our world was expanding, and that people were accepting us as a couple. That was the best feeling in the world. At her party I was treated as wonderfully as she was. Her parents even got a special ice cream cake for me, which I loved. At times I felt like pinching myself to see if it was real, because I could not believe how well I was treated.

Though my school year progressed just the same way, I will admit that most of my studies took a backseat to Alex and my music. If I could not be with Alex, I would be singing or listening to music. If I could not do any of those, I was restless. I often lost interest in my classes, but somehow was able to focus enough to maintain good grades. This was important because it kept the adults off my back and allowed me much more freedom to be with the person that I loved.

By the time Christmas rolled around, Alex and I were already making plans for a big family celebration that would include both our families getting together. This was also my first Christmas with Alex, and that alone was the best present that anyone could ever receive.

Even though we were still teens, the holidays felt more like a coming together of families, the kind you have when you get engaged. Everyone worries about whether or not their folks will get along with the other person's folks. Everyone wants desperately to please everyone else, make all the others happy and have everything go smoothly. I am happy to say that it went even better than that. Our families spent most of the day together and it was another magical one for both of us.

Another highlight of the day, besides having Alex by my side, and parking my chair directly under the mistletoe, was one special present that I received: my first guitar. Though Alex was still my main focus in life, my guitar would soon become an important part of my world, and something that also helped to save my life.

Chapter Twenty-Four: The Prom

The highlight of the entire school year (and my life) was soon approaching. I was a junior and everyone knows what that means: Junior Prom. When I heard the first announcement at school, I immediately thought back to the awkward days of Junior High dances and how I felt like such an outsider. But I didn't let that influence my decision one bit. When I heard those words, I knew that I was going and I was taking Alex with me.

I can remember telling Mom about it. Her reaction was predictable.

"Hey, Mom, good news!" I said one evening.

"What's that?" she asked. "You get 100 on your math test?"

"Not quite," I replied, knowing by her smirk that she was probably teasing me. "The Junior Prom is going to be held in May."

"And?" she said, stringing me along.

"And I want to go?"

"Is that all?" she continued.

"Is that all? Um, no. I want to take Alex with me. I want us both to go to the prom!"

"Is that all?" she asked again.

"Well, yeah, I guess. That's all. I want us to go to the Prom."

"OK," Mom said. "You just let me know what you need and I will make sure it gets done."

"I guess I will need something to wear. Alex, too. And maybe flowers. And transportation. I'm not sure."

"OK. We'll make it work. I promise."

I promise. Just like that. It was just that easy. And I knew that she meant every word that she said. When Mom said something would get done, it got done. The only thing left were the details. Mom had it all under control.

Mom helped to coordinate our wardrobes. Alex was to wear a lime green dress that perfectly complimented her blonde hair and made her look so grown up. I was color-coordinated with Alex, and was to be dressed in a white tuxedo with a green vest.

The day of the prom came, and I was nervous. Mom took Alex to get her hair done, while I got scrubbed cleaner than I had ever been my entire life. I was polished to perfection, smelling sweet and looking good as I sat in my chair and waited for Alex to make her entrance. And what an entrance that was! She was more beautiful than I had ever seen her, or anyone else for that matter. She was like a vision as she walked into my living room and made her way toward me. Her face was glowing like the sun itself. She was perfection. If we had just met for the first time, right at that very second, I would have fallen in love with her on the spot.

Alex came to me and kissed me on the cheek. The magical

night had begun.

Our carriage awaited, but in our case, the carriage was my van. My folks chauffeured us around, making us feel like stars. Our first stop was at my parents' friends' house to have our pictures taken in the lovely, scenic spot by the water. After that, we headed off to an elegant restaurant to share a wonderful dinner. The final stop was the Prom.

My parents dropped us off, told us they would be back later, and left. We were, for the most part, on our own. As we entered the room and saw all of our friends, I could not help but be impressed by the fanciness of it all. It was dark and sophisticated with colored lights glimmering. It seemed like everything sparkled.

All my friends were there, dressed up in clothes that made them hard to recognize. What a change from the shorts and t-shirts they wore to school. Some of these kids actually looked good! Though the guys were dressed better than I had ever seen them before, the girls looked even better. The beauty in that room was astounding. Yet, I could not help but think to myself that I was so lucky to be there with the best-looking girl of them all.

We milled around for a while, talking to people and having photos taken. Some people danced and others sat at tables. The music was loud, and the place began to rock. All of a sudden, I did not feel so good anymore. I looked around at all of the others who were dancing, and thoughts of awkward and uncomfortable Junior High dances flashed into my memory.

My mood must have been written all over my face, because Alex noticed it in a flash.

"What's the matter, Baby?" she asked.

"Nothing," I replied, trying to hide it as best I could.

207

"Come on, something's wrong. I can tell. I can see it. You can't hide it from me. What's wrong, Honey? Tell me."

I didn't want to admit it, but it was one of the few times of my life when I felt frustrated because I could not do something. It was the first time that I felt less than everyone else. It was the first time that I wished my legs could work enough so that I could stand up and dance with my girl. But how could I admit that to her without appearing less of a man?

"I…I…" I stammered.

"Tell me, Baby."

"I want to dance with you," I admitted, tears now starting to well up in my eyes.

"Aw, Honey," Alex said. "If you want to dance, then let's dance."

"But…"

"There's no way I'm not going to dance with my man," she added.

"But, how?"

Alex stood right in front of me. She leaned closer and kissed me right in front of everyone. And, though the music was probably still playing, in my mind it stopped. All of a sudden the room froze and it was only the two of us in the entire place.

Alex began to carefully loosen the straps that held me in place on my wheelchair. She loosened my head brace, and my head slowly tilted toward her. She gently held it so as not to move too far forward. Then she undid the straps that held my chest upright in the chair. She slowly slid me forward until I was close enough so that she could wrap her arms around me in an embrace.

There we were, on the dance floor, holding one another. The music began to grow louder and we began to sway to it, slowly and gently. We were dancing.

Alex then whispered into my ear, "How's this, Baby?"

"Perfect. Just perfect," I said.

And I meant every word of it.

"I love you, Craig."

"I love you, Alexandra."

And I meant every word of that, too.

PICTURES

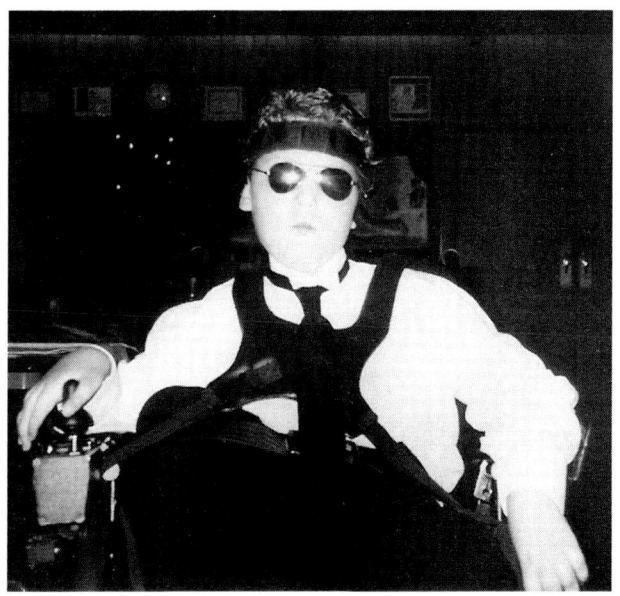

This is my cool look. How do you like the sunglasses?

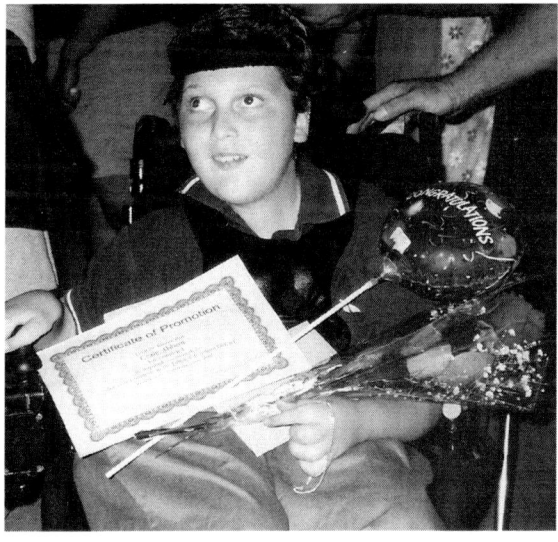

This is me at my elementary school graduation.

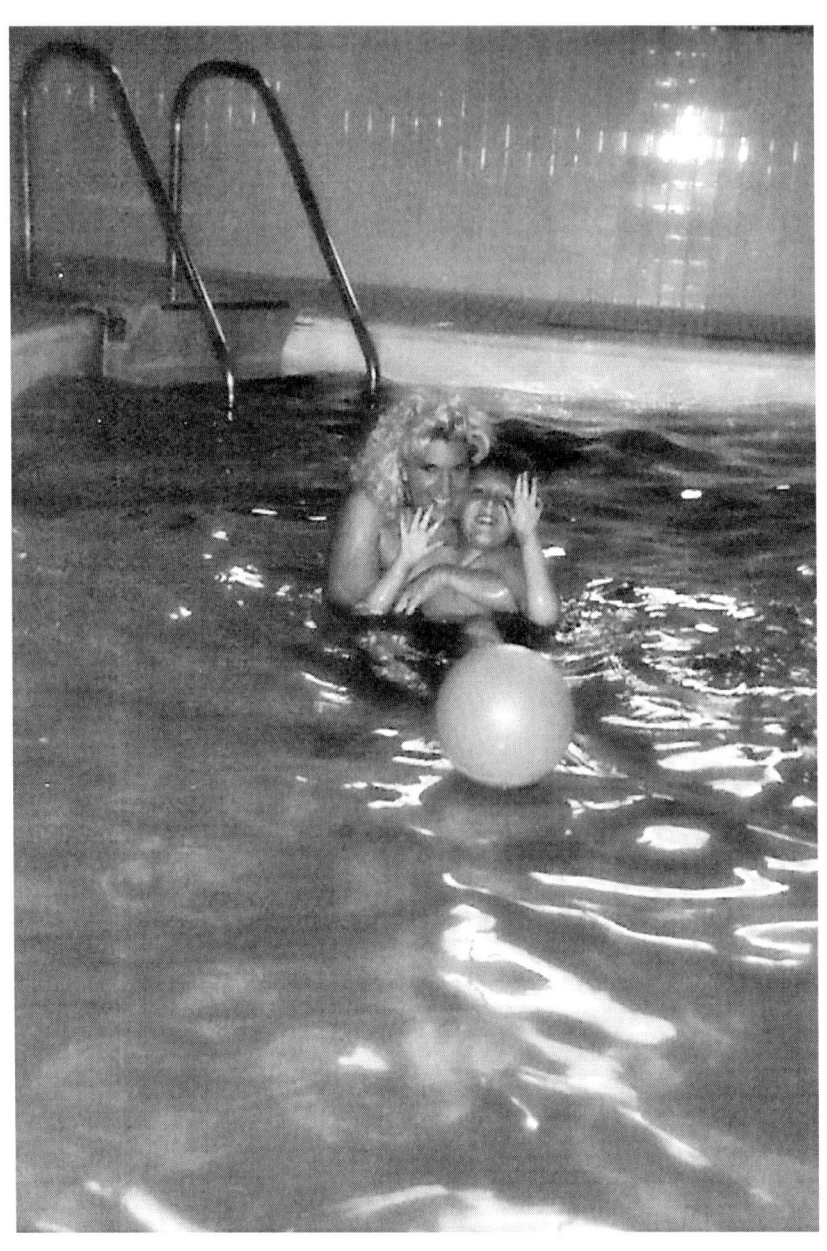

One of my favorites – me with Mom!

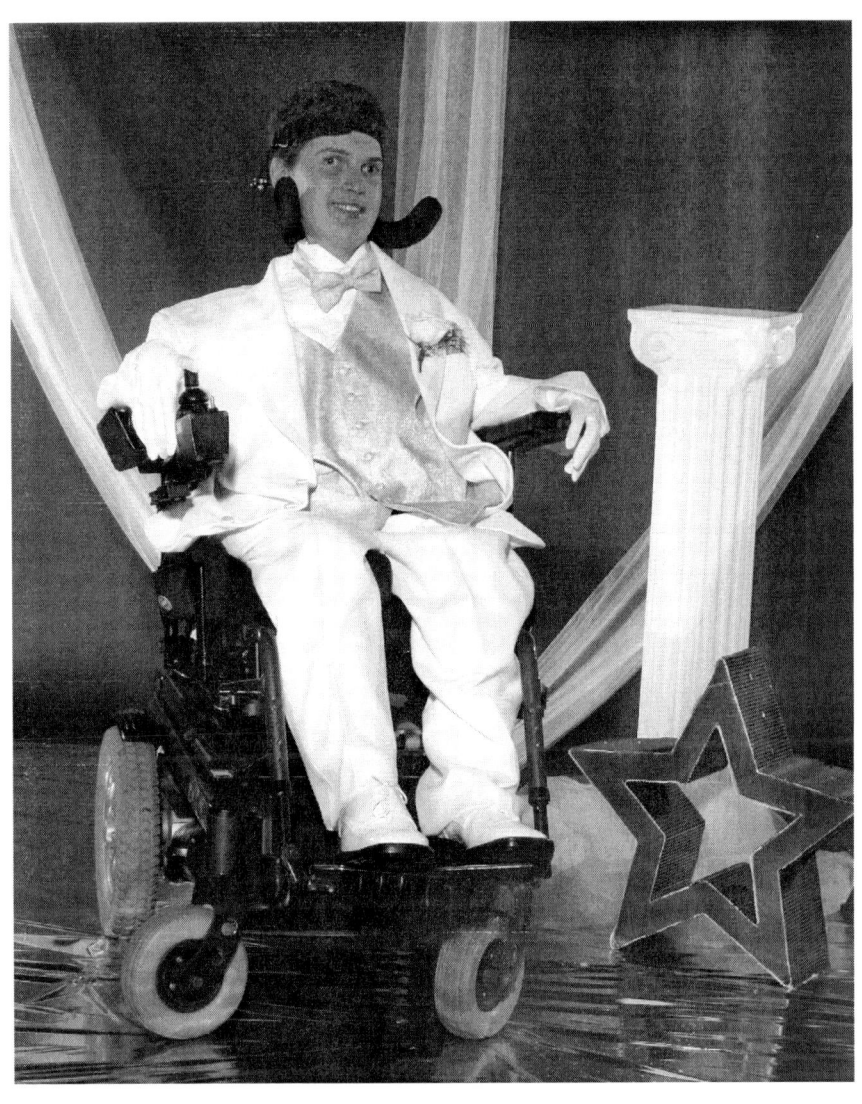

My high school prom picture. May, 2006.

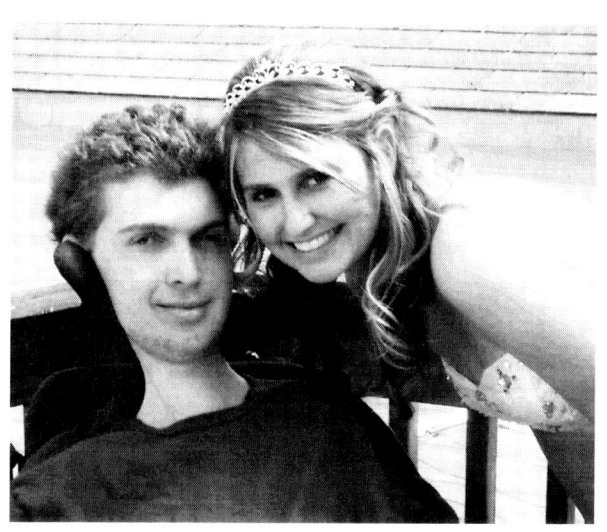

My best friend – my sister Cralynne.

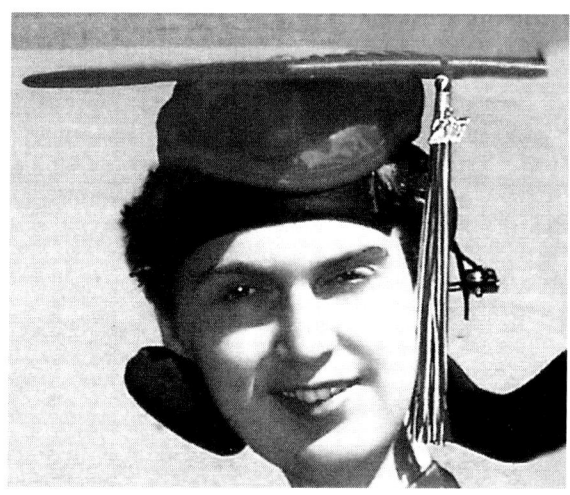

High School Graduation: G. Ray Bodley High School, Fulton,
New York, June 2007.

They said I would never make it, but I graduated right on time, right
alongside all my classmates and friends.

Chapter Twenty-Five: Explosion

If my life could have ended the morning after the Junior Prom, I would have died a happy man. I would have gone out on top, just like a quarterback who retires after leading his team to a Super Bowl victory or a starting pitcher after winning game 7 of the World Series. It's good to go out on top, instead of watching things slowly slip away, while you try in futile exhaustion to desperately get back to where you once were.

It wasn't that I was feeling down after the Prom had ended. On the contrary, it was just the opposite. In my mind, the perfect days would continue. In my mind, Alex and I would always be together. I always thought it was a done deal. And since our relationship in the days that followed was as good as ever, what did I have to worry about?

Junior year ended on a high note. One day, during final exams week, my math teacher told me that he had a gift for me. I was overwhelmed. I had never heard of a teacher giving a present to a student. I thought it was the other way around.

He proceeded to give me a really cool, black electric bass

guitar. He wanted me to try playing bass because he felt that might be easier for me to accomplish. He knew how much I loved music, and he wanted me to keep going. I guess he could tell that I hadn't given playing the guitar a good shot. He knew that my first attempts to play the guitar were a struggle.

I did seek help in the form of a guitar instructor, but that didn't turn out well. My instructor had been discouraging and negative. He had an "Are you kidding me?" attitude that rubbed me the wrong way. He was of the opinion that I could never learn how to play – and he said so to my face. Others had tried to help, including Alex, but none of them yielded the results I had hoped for. Teaching myself to play was the only option left.

I could not thank my math teacher enough for the generous gift. But even though I was excited about the guitar and I wanted to continue with my music, I could not spare the time. I had no place for it in my world. All that I had room for was Alex. So I put the guitar on hold for a while.

Summer finally arrived and that meant I no longer had to waste my time in boring classes. I could now spend every waking moment with Alex. Alex felt even stronger about it. She never wanted to leave my side – ever. This often led to awkward discussions between her and my nurses. You see, Alex soon wanted to do everything for me. She wanted to become my nurse.

The nurses had mixed feelings about this. Some felt that this was fine – treating her just like a family member learning how to care for me. They would go so far as to teach her what to do. But others weren't so keen on the idea, citing her age and inexperience as a potentially dangerous problem. But I will say this in Alex's defense: she never once made a mistake. When she learned how to do something, she did it correctly. I was never in jeopardy when I was in her caring hands.

Early that summer, my family felt that a vacation away from home might do us some good. Of course I told everyone that the vacation had to include Alex or I simply would not go. They agreed to my demands, so the whole bunch of us – Alex, Cralynne, my nurse, my parents and myself – all jumped into the van and motored off to Niagara Falls. It was a wonderful time. Then again, any time with Alex was destined to be wonderful.

For the most part, the remainder of the summer was good. Alex and I spent a lot of time babysitting her cousins. It was fun to pretend that someday this would be just how life would be for us. It was fun to imagine that we had our own home and were busy raising our own family. We even added a few pets into the equation, as we both loved animals. One day we brought a kitten home and adopted it as our own. And we purchased some geckos that we kept in a large terrarium in my living area. Our family was expanding and we loved it.

Unfortunately, I was once again struggling with my health that summer. And although I could have looked at another run of ill health as a setback, I never did. That is the wrong way to approach life. Every life has bumps along the way. It's best to tackle them head-first, fight back hard, learn what you can from the experience, and then move on. Dwelling on adversity, sitting back and moaning with a "why me" attitude accomplishes nothing. It is a total waste of time.

Alex felt the same way. She had always been a "jump right in there" type of person. She never let life slow her down or get in her way. When faced with a problem, she would hardly let a second pass before she was figuring out ways to solve it. That was another thing that I loved about her.

By time, Alex knew how to run all of my machines. She knew what needed to be done to keep me healthy. If anyone thought she was always at my side when I was healthy, well they should have seen her when I was ill. You could not pry her away from me. When I would become congested, Alex would use my Cough Assist to help clear my lungs. When I had difficulties, she would pound on my chest in order to help loosen the congestion until her small hands were raw. And when I was coughing and gagging and struggling to breathe, she was right by my side, hands covered with my phlegm as I coughed it up. She would clean me up afterwards, never complaining, always smiling. What an angel!

I suppose that the only problem with Alex's nurturing nature is the controlling aspect of it. Instead of jumping in and helping alongside of everyone else, Alex wanted them out of the way. She wanted to be my sole protector and savior. She had a hard time letting others get close to me. Tension started to build between Alex and the other people close to me, though at the time, I was blind to any of this. I didn't even realize the obsessive nature that our relationship was taking when she spoke about keeping my friends away from me. All that I could see was that I had the most beautiful and wonderful girl in the world all to myself; and if that meant building a wall around us, so be it.

We survived the summer and that meant the inevitable was upon us. School had to start. Neither one of us was looking forward to once again being robbed of our "together time." We wished that we could speed up the clock and be done with school for good. We wanted to be out on our own, married, and raising a family. Our relationship was evolving – some said it was out of control – and the world was not keeping pace with us.

In fairness, we were both becoming obsessed with our relationship, but in different ways. Since our personalities were remarkably similar in nature, it was easy to see eye-to-eye with how we should deal with the rest of the world. But when one of us wanted to exercise a little control over the other, well, look out!

I recall one day when Alex decided to pull a little surprise on me that I did not like one bit. It was early one morning and my Grandpa had parked the van in front of Alex's house. The two of us sat and waited for her to get in. As the door opened and she climbed inside, my mouth dropped open.

"What the hell did you to do your hair?" I tactfully blurted out.

"I colored it," Alex answered as she took her place beside me.

"I can see that," I replied.

"Then why did you ask?" she shot back at me.

"OK. OK. How's this? Why the hell did you dye your hair brown?"

"I thought it might look good. I thought I could use the change."

"It doesn't and you don't," I explained angrily. "Change it back."

"Why?"

"Because I hate it."

"What about me? What if I like it?"

"But it's brown!"

"So?" she asked defiantly.

"So, I hate it!"

"It's my hair," she explained.

219

"So?" I asked defiantly.

"So, don't I get a say in the matter?" she continued.

"No…er…yes…I mean, I don't know. That's not the point."

"What is the point?"

I paused for a second. This wasn't getting us anywhere. I needed to collect my thoughts so I could persuade her to do the right thing.

"OK, look," I said, "Yes, it is your hair, and yes, you do have the right to color it whatever you want…red…orange…blue…"

She started to smile. I was winning her over.

"But the point is, it doesn't look good on you," I explained.

"Maybe I should get some other opinions. Maybe I should ask some other guys what they think…"

"No! No other guys. Stay away from guys."

"Why?"

"Because they'll just lie to you and say it looks fine. They'll just…oh, never mind. Just trust me."

"Trust you?"

"Babe, you had the most beautiful blonde hair I have ever seen, the most beautiful blonde hair on the planet. Why change? Nothing could ever look as good. Nothing. Ever. Trust me."

"But I thought you might like the change."

"I never want anything to change. Ever. Unless it would mean that we could be closer."

Alex smiled her alluring smile, her sparkling white teeth beaming from beneath her hideous brown mane.

"What do you say? Will you change it back?" I asked.

"It's not that easy," she explained.

"For me?" I pleaded

OK," she conceded. "For you."

Disaster averted.

That little spat wasn't the only rough patch that we went through, though we never noticed what was coming. They say that love is blind; and now I know what they meant. We were headed for disaster at the speed of light; completely unaware of what was happening.

I started becoming more distracted at school with every passing day. It's not that my classes were boring, it's that everything was boring in comparison to Alex. I did not want to do anything but be with her. As a result, I did the minimum amount of work that I could, just enough to keep my grades up. Still, my time apart from Alex was spent in a perpetual daydream. Whenever I had the chance, I would slip away into our perfect world and stay there until the slap of reality brought me back to the mundane.

Sometimes when we were apart, I would sit and wonder what Alex was doing. I would imagine her in class, the center of attention, answering all the questions correctly, making everyone envious of her intelligence, making the girls jealous of her beauty, and making the boys want to be with her. Then I got angry. The thought of other guys trying to make a move made my skin crawl. When it came to girls, I did not like competition. Alex was mine.

221

Unfortunately, Alex felt the same way about me. And it wasn't just that she did not like girls paying attention to me. She didn't like *anyone* paying attention to me. That even included my family and friends. Pretty soon, it got to the point where Alex did not want me to see my friends anymore. I began making excuses why I couldn't do things with them or why they could not come to the house. Even my cousin, David, who I still saw on occasion, had to go through the trouble of calling first and then sneaking in and out of my house, just to make sure Alex did not catch him. He had to do all that just to see me. Call it what you will: ridiculous, unfair, hurtful. It was what I put people through, just so I could be with my girl. I am very ashamed at all of it now, but as it happened I accepted every bit of it as being completely fine. I thought our relationship was stronger and healthier than ever. I completely lost touch with the rest of the world.

Day by day, the wall that we were building around us was turning into a fortress. No one was allowed in without permission. We had done it. We had shut everyone else out. Friends did not come around anymore. My nurses were alienated and only performed whatever tasks they could manage. More and more they had to spend time outside of my living area, sitting and waiting all day just in case I would call upon them. But I never did anymore. Alex took care of everything.

My family was shut out as well. We were passing strangers in a cold, uncomfortable house. I never spoke to anyone, opting instead for more and more time with Alex, who just about lived with me by then. Even my mom was becoming alienated from me. That is what finally did it. That is what caused our wall to come tumbling down.

I should have seen it coming all along. People were always trying to give me advice. Mom was always suggesting that I see other people, hang out with my friends once again, or even take a break

222

from Alex. I ignored every single word. I had to. Alex had become like a drug to me and I could not get enough of her.

Then came the day when Mom put her foot down.

"Craig, I want you to stop seeing Alex for a while," she said.

"What? No way. Are you joking?" I asked.

"No, I think you need a break from one another," she explained.

"A break? Why do we need a break? Everything is perfect, Mom. We love each other."

"Everything is not perfect. You just can't see it because you're in love."

"Yes, we're in love. We're totally in love. And what's wrong with that?" I asked, as I was starting to feel threatened.

"Nothing's wrong with being in love. Being in love is wonderful. But even when you're in love, your life has to have some balance. You can't just be in love and stop living."

"Stop living? Mom, you're being ridiculous. I have never felt more alive!"

"I know that's how you feel inside, but just look at you. Look at what you've become."

"What have I become? I am happy and I am in love. I have found my woman. What have I become? I've become a man!"

"But look at how you treat everyone else," Mom continued.

"I don't care about anyone else!"

223

Mom continued lecturing me and I grew agitated. I began playing with the controller on my chair, fidgeting back and forth, and wanting to escape, wanting to run off and be with Alex.

"Craig, this relationship is not healthy. You need time to back off a bit and think about what is going on with this girl."

"This girl? This girl? Her name is Alex, Mom. Don't ever call her this girl again. Alex is a woman and I love her."

"Alex is 16."

"So? What's wrong with that? You're not being fair. People can be grown up at 16. You're not talking about kids here. You're talking about two people who are in love and who want to be together for the rest of their lives."

"No, it's too soon to decide all of that. You're so young. You have so much ahead of you."

"All I want ahead of me is Alex! That is all that I want."

"And what about the rest of the world?" Mom asked.

"The rest of the world can just kiss my…"

"Craig! Stop!"

There was silence for a second. I wanted to yell, but felt like I should stay quiet. I was angry and confused. I felt like I had been ambushed. Then Mom delivered the crushing blow.

"This has got to stop and this has got to stop now. I am putting my foot down. You can't have people sneaking in and out just to see you. You can't just forget about school and your future. This is not a healthy way to live and it has got to change. So I am forbidding you from seeing Alex."

"You can't," I shot back.

"Yes, I can," Mom replied. "And I will."

"No, Mom, no!"

"I'm sorry, but it's for your own good."

"No, Mom!"

"I've made my decision and that's that. I forbid you from going to her house, and I forbid her from coming here. And you can't date her again until I say so."

"No, Mom!"

"I'm going to make sure everyone knows so that there won't be any way that you can sneak off and see her. No one is going to help you. The relationship is off limits. You can't see Alex anymore."

"You can't make me!" I yelled.

"Oh yes I can!" Mom yelled back. Then she left.

I let out a scream that I am sure the neighbors heard. I felt like my heart had been ripped out of my chest. It hurt. It hurt so bad. It hurt worse than any disease or trip to the hospital or operation. It felt like I was dead inside.

There have been a few rare times when I cursed my situation. There have been a few times that I wished I could have gotten up out of my chair and done things. But none of those times can compare to what I was feeling at that moment. The reason that it hurt so much is because I knew Mom was right. I knew that she could stop me. I knew that she could have everyone keep Alex out of the house. I knew that she could tell people to keep an eye on me. And I knew that if no one would help me get out of the house, into my van, and over to wherever Alex was, I was powerless on my own. I began to cry.

Mom had managed to take the woman that I loved out of my life. She had managed to rob me of everything that I ever wanted. Both my room and my heart were dark and empty. The wall that we had built was now my prison. I might have just as well been dead.

I cried endlessly after that, clinging on to the slim hope that Mom would either change her mind or slip up. It never happened. She was just too competent to make a stupid mistake. She managed to keep Alex away from me.

As soon as Alex found out, she came over to my house. Although I never got to see her, I heard her voice outside. I have been told that she confronted my mother, wanting to know why things had to be this way. It must have been just as puzzling to her as it was to me when I heard the news. It must have hurt her just as much as it hurt me.

The voices were muffled. I could not make out the words. But I heard some yelling. People were angry. At first I tried to get closer, but my nurse reminded me that I had better not. I would have tried to force my way out of the house, except that I realized it wouldn't do any good. It might have made it worse. If anyone could convince my mother to do something, it would be Alex.

But she didn't. She couldn't. Mom was firm in her stand. We had no choice in the matter. The grown-ups had won.

When the voices stopped, I grew hopeful. I had wild visions of Alex and my mom walking through the door, smiling, arms wrapped around each other. There was no such luck.

My mom walked in all by herself, looked me straight in the eye and said, "Alex won't be coming over anymore."

It was over.

Mom's plan worked. There was no hope of contacting Alex. The only time I saw her was in passing at school. The first time, my heart sank. I had tears in my eyes. I wanted to call out, but my nurse was with me. I was helpless to do anything. After that, we just turned our heads away from one another because the pain was unbearable. I felt completely numb inside; and I am sure she did, too.

After that – I have no idea for how long – things were just a blur. While the plan worked in keeping us apart, it did not work at getting me to do anything else. I went to school because I had to. The rest of the time, I sulked or cried. I did a lot of crying, for weeks and weeks and weeks. That's all there was. Then, I found the one thing that stopped me from hitting rock bottom: I rediscovered my music.

I don't know why this happened, but one day I asked my nurse to hand me my guitar. She placed it in my lap and I stared at it for a while. I slowly ran my hand up the neck. I felt the curve of its body. I knew exactly what I had to do. If I could not make love to my girl, I was going to make love to my guitar.

It wasn't easy at first. I was still very new at it and I faced challenges; the biggest of which being how in the world could I ever manage the logistics of getting my fingers into the positions needed to play. I had to devise my own system of playing the guitar if this was going to work. I had to invent something.

There was no way that I could ever play the guitar the same way that everyone else did. It was simply impossible. First of all, I could not hold it. I did not have the strength to do it. This was simple to fix. I could have the guitar placed across my lap and play it the same way that they play a steel guitar in a country band. The first time I realized this, I chuckled. *Well, they finally did it,* I thought. *They finally got me to play country-style.*

A pillow was placed on my lap. Then my guitar was set on top of that, positioned so that I could strum with my right hand and use my left hand for fingering.

The next problem that I faced was the most serious of all: fingering. My fingers are almost useless in terms of dexterity, flexibility, and strength. I can use them a bit, but it is always a struggle. So how could I ever manage to manipulate them and press down hard enough onto the metal strings to play the chords? It looked impossible. And it was – if you approach it the "normal" way. So I had to approach it in "my normal" way.

I decided that, while I could not get my fingertips into place, I could get my fingers to cooperate if I folded the fingers in, looking almost like I was making a fist, and then pressing onto the strings with my second finger joints, the ones between the first joints and the knuckles. It looked weird, but it worked. The only problem with doing that was that it was impossible to stretch my hand enough to reach all the strings. But I fixed that problem, too.

I changed the way the strings were tuned. Instead of the traditional E,A,D,G,B,E method, I tuned my strings to be C,G,C,F,A,D. This allowed me to be able to hit the notes I needed in the chords I wanted to play. If I pressed down with all my might, I could use my finger joints and thumb to make music. I had a plan!

I tore into that guitar the same way that I tore into life: relentlessly. I spent all my waking hours pouring out my pain into those six strings. My fingers became raw and bruised and, sometimes, bloody because I refused to take it slow. And I refused to stop because, when I stopped, I felt too much pain. It felt better to express it. My weak arms grew sore as hour after hour I strained to press down. My guitar became my new obsession. My guitar was my savior and my love.

The remainder of my senior year can be easily painted with a gray brush. Classes were a mere formality, as we counted down the days to graduation. Though I did start to reconnect with my friends, there was no place for female companionship in my life. Alex and I were kept apart. The only way to survive was not to think about it. As soon as thoughts turned to Alex, the pain returned, as strong as ever, and my emotions had to be released on my guitar.

Graduation came, and I did manage a few smiles, especially when I saw how happy everyone was for me. People said that I had beaten the odds. I would say more accurately, that I had crushed them. But I really don't look at it that way. When people tell me that, it's like they are saying, "Oh, you poor guy to have all this bad stuff happen to you. You did great!" But that is pity and I don't want pity. Never once did I doubt that I could get through school. Never once did I doubt that I could learn to play the guitar. Never once did I doubt that I could do anything.

I graduated with honors, and was all set to start college in the fall. The promise of higher education was ahead of me. It was supposed to be a happy time, but it wasn't. I still felt the void of life without Alex. I feel it to this very day. With college ahead, there was hope of a new tomorrow. Only I wasn't sure whether my future was bright or not. I wasn't sure where my life was heading.

Chapter Twenty-Six: Biding My Time

It was the summer that I was to turn eighteen: when people finally look at you as an adult, the age when people finally take you seriously. I was fresh out of high school and headed for college. Doors were opening up for me. It was a time when I should have felt on top of the world. So why didn't I?

My life was a total state of confusion. I wanted to go to college, but I wasn't sure what I wanted to study. I wanted a girlfriend, but if it couldn't be Alex, what was the point? Nothing seemed right. I could not get motivated. I could not figure things out. I wasn't myself.

I felt as if someone had placed me in a spin dryer and turned it up to full speed. Each and every thought that entered my head was followed by another thought that contradicted it, tore it apart, and left me bewildered. I had big decisions to make; and here I was feeling like a complete idiot. If somebody asked me what I felt like doing that day, I would answer "shoe." That's how confused I was. I was an alien in my own world, my own town, my own skin. I was trapped with no way out in sight.

People started to notice that the boy who always smiled wasn't smiling. Everyone tried to help, but as far as I was concerned, it was just more advice that I didn't want.

Cralynne tried to help cheer me up by telling jokes, something that we used to do a lot. I guess she felt that a few jokes would help me start showing off the old pearly whites again, something that she always did. I think Cralynne smiled even more than I did. But it didn't work. All that it did was leave her frustrated – yet still smiling as usual.

Grandpa hoped to distract me by trying to get me more interested in music. That didn't help either. By that time, our tastes had grown so far apart it was like we were on opposite ends of the Grand Canyon. Grandpa likes religious music. I like heavy metal. The two of us were never going to agree on anything musical. It was a disaster. In fact, he didn't like anything that wasn't religious. Even country music was too wild for him. According to Grandpa, "It's either Jesus music or it's not!" Case closed.

I usually followed our discussions by spending some alone time with Metallica blasted as loud as I could manage without getting into trouble. That made me feel better…until the music stopped. After that, it was just spiral back into my dark and unhappy place.

Mom thought I could snap out of it simply by doing things and keeping constantly busy. I think she underestimated the depths of my sadness and confusion. I think she didn't realize how much I still missed Alex.

"Craig, you need to get out more," she would tell me, over and over."

"Yes, Mom, I know."

"Get out of the house. Go someplace. Do something. Get a new perspective on things."

I had heard the advice a million times. It wasn't going to work.

"You'll see. As soon as you get out of the house, everything will seem better. You'll be yourself in no time."

I began to wonder how long "no time" was. It was well over six months since she split Alex and me apart. Well over six months, and I had been out of the house many times. So what was one more trip to the mall going to do? Cheer me up? Was I supposed to get excited because there was a sale on hoodies at Old Navy? It wasn't that simple. Nothing was simple anymore.

Even my friends began to grow frustrated with me. They would still visit the house. They would still want to do things with me. But I just moped and they eventually left, shaking their heads in disbelief and frustration.

J.T. was especially aggravated by my behavior. He thought he knew what was wrong with me. He might have been the closest to getting it right.

"Bro, you have got to snap out of this," J.T. would say.

"I'm fine," I would always snap back.

"Don't give me that. You're not fine."

"I'm fine."

"Don't treat me like I'm stupid. You're not fine. I can see it. Everyone can see it."

"I'm fine."

"Well, if that's what you believe, you're in denial," J.T. said.

"Fine. I'm in denial," I shot back. "But I still don't wanna go for a ride. I don't wanna go to the mall. I don't wanna look at guitars or new music."

"Who said anything about going to the mall, Bro? That's not what's wrong. That's not what you need."

"OK, Einstein, what do I need?"

"A female. A woman. A babe," J.T. answered. "You need to go on a date. You need a girlfriend."

I didn't reply because I felt that he had hit the nail on the head. It was too soon to think about another girl. Even if I needed another girl, I didn't want one if it wasn't Alex. It made me feel angry that people underestimated our love. It made me feel angry that people did not realize the pain that ripping us apart caused. It made me feel like no one respected our feelings.

"I'm fine," I answered, figuring that being in denial was better than opening up old wounds.

"OK, Bro, whatever," J.T. said. "Just remember that whenever you decide that it's time to jump back into the babe pool, I got your back."

I nodded and that was the end of the discussion.

J.T. was right. I knew it. I was lacking female companionship. I missed having a woman around. Still, as I said, if it wasn't going to be Alex, then why even bother?

One thing I noticed about having a relationship with the opposite sex is that, given enough time, the brain stops thinking. You need it. You crave it. And sooner or later logic and wisdom take a vacation in favor of hormones and lust. This is precisely what happened to me, even though I tried my best to prevent it, even though I told myself over and over not to ever ask anyone out because they could never measure up to Alex.

Her name was Chelsea; and we had met, of all places, at church. My wandering eye had caught sight of her one Sunday while Grandpa was busy belting out some Jesus music. We met and had chatted several times, so we weren't exactly strangers, just polite acquaintances.

Chelsea was a little younger than Alex, but the two were in the same grade. She was on the short side, with one of the sweetest and most innocent faces that I had ever seen. She had auburn hair, and I think that is what attracted me to her so much. Since she seemed very different from Alex, I thought that a relationship might be possible because I wouldn't compare the two of them.

I had finally decided that enough was enough. I had been without a female by my side way too long. I called Chelsea, and we hit it off right away. I asked her out and she did not hesitate in saying "yes." Another relationship had started.

Chelsea and I began dating as the summer unfolded. At first, she would most often come to my place and hang out with me. But soon I got the feeling that it made her uncomfortable to be there. She didn't like to look at all my machines and my medicine. If something happened and my nurse had to help me, Chelsea would do her best to look the other way or leave the room. I got the feeling that she had a hard time coming to terms with my illness. But I didn't care. I had a woman near me again.

As a result of how Chelsea felt about the machines that surrounded my bed, we started spending a lot of time away from my house. Sometimes we would walk down to my park, meet up with friends, or just hang out and watch the kids have fun. I enjoyed spending time there because it reminded me how I had beaten the odds. It reminded me that it was OK not to listen what doctors said if that meant you had to give up. It made me feel good to be there.

235

We also spent a lot of time at the mall. Chelsea loved the mall. I didn't mind it, either. The mall was always full of people, mostly young people. There were plenty of places to go, plenty of stores to browse through, and plenty of women to gaze at. What's not to like?

Though we did spend many an hour roaming through the crowd of bored young people with too much time on their hands, we had differing thoughts about what stores to visit. Chelsea liked to look at clothes – woman's clothes. I didn't. The only good thing about spending any time at all in a woman's clothing store was getting Chelsea to model for me. I didn't mind that one bit. It didn't feel too bad when the end result was a fashion show.

I, on the other hand, preferred the music store and the video game shop. No big surprise. One of the few places that we had in common was any store that sold hoodies. I loved my hoodies and could never get enough of them. That and Dunkin' Donuts. I loved my coffee, too. Still do. But no matter how you look at it, trips to the mall were always an exercise in compromise.

"Okay, where do you wanna go?" was Chelsea's inevitable first question.

"Music store. Where else?" I would always reply. This was always followed by her slight sigh of disappointment.

"Do we have to?" she would ask.

"Um…yeah! What good is a trip to the mall without checking out the music?"

"But I want to look for something for the beach," she'd explain.

"Cool, let's find some new music for the beach."

"OK, smart guy, you know what I meant."

I did, but I wasn't going to admit it.

"I need to try on clothes," she'd say.

"Need? Does anybody really need to do that?"

"Yes, we do, unless you want everyone to be naked."

I just smiled. Chelsea got the message.

"OK, how about we go to the music store and then I try on clothes? I'll model for you again."

That almost did it. Not quite.

"How about we hit up Dunkin' Donuts first. I need a latte," I added.

"Does anybody really need a latte?" she countered.

"I do!"

And that was that, because Chelsea knew that I really needed one. Having now planned out our mall adventure, we embarked on our date.

One of the advantages to dating Chelsea was that she liked to go places. That meant that I would tag along, get out of the house, and escape the funk that I had seemingly been in forever. We spent a lot of time at her place, too. I went to her family's barbeques and get-togethers all throughout the summer. And that is where I met one of my closest friends, Chelsea's brother, Johnny.

Johnny impressed me right from the start. And why not? When you are six foot seven you are impressive. He had short, straight hair, more of a strawberry blonde color, but you couldn't always see it because he liked to wear a cap and a hoodie over that…even in the summer. Pretty impressive.

Johnny was very much like me in one special way. He liked to be active. Johnny loved riding motorcycles, dirt bikes, and anything that went fast. So did I, only I couldn't. The only thing that I could do was to crank up the accelerator on my chair as high as it would go, or yell at my grandpa to drive the van a lot faster.

I suppose that you could say that I lived vicariously through Johnny. I know that sounds sad, but it isn't. The reality of it is that I have always known what was impossible for me to do; and I have accepted that with no regrets. I got just as big a thrill seeing Johnny pop a wheelie on a motorcycle as I would if I had done it myself. Well, almost.

Soon Johnny and I were best friends. He became like a big brother to me. He liked to think that he protected me – not that I needed protecting. I could take care of myself when push came to shove. But Johnny's protective nature – and size – made me feel even more fearless because he was like my bodyguard. Nobody was going to mess with me when Johnny was around. Did I mention that he was impressive?

Our relationship grew stronger over time. It was clear that it was going to last. Unfortunately, I cannot say the same thing about Chelsea and me. Toward the end of the summer, we started having troubles.

It all began innocently one evening. Chelsea had spent the day with me, and we were just starting to relax at my place for some private time. We were alone and things were starting to get physical. We shared a kiss and an embrace. Chelsea began caressing me in a more serious manner. She moved even closer.

My heart began to race…not in a good way. My mind was traveling in a million directions all at once. I could not understand why this did not feel good to me, why it bothered me. I could not understand why I wanted her to stop. Here I was alone in my room with a beautiful girl, and I wanted her to stop. I thought I had lost my mind.

The more it progressed, the worse it got. I flashed back to all those intimate moments with Alex, and how right they felt. My heart started to ache for her once again. Something deep inside kept saying "This is wrong. This is wrong."

I tried to fight it as best I could. I wanted to be close to Chelsea. I needed to be close to Chelsea. But I couldn't.

Faster and faster my heart pounded. My breathing became strained. I started gasping for air. My skin grew sweaty. The room began to darken as I felt light-headed. My first thought was that I was having a heart attack.

Chelsea nuzzled my neck, and I felt like I could no longer breathe. I needed help. I couldn't take it.

"Call 911! Call 911!"I screamed.

Chelsea jumped back from me. Her face turned completely white.

"What's the matter, Craig?" she yelled. "What's wrong?"

"I can't breathe. Call 911. I have to go to the hospital!"

Chelsea began to cry. She started to run out of the room, just as my nurse was running in. My nurse looked at me gasping for air and immediately got onto the phone.

"Hang on, C.V.!" she said. "They're coming. An ambulance

will be here soon. Just hang on."

My nurse started checking my vital signs and tried to comfort me as Chelsea stood in the corner horrified. She never spoke a word. She looked like she wanted to run away from the whole episode.

My nurse didn't ask questions. She knew what was going on. It's a good thing, because if she did, I am certain that Chelsea would have completely panicked.

"Hang on, C.V. Just a little longer. They'll be here soon. Try and stay calm. Try to take short breaths. It won't be long now."

"It won't be long? It won't be long?" I thought. *"What does she mean? Am I dying? Does she know that I am dying? What in the world is happening to me? Somebody please help me. I can't breathe!"*

Soon I heard the drone of the siren and I knew that help was on the way. I was again whisked off to the Emergency Room at Lee Memorial Hospital, and my all-too-familiar journey had begun again.

I wish that I could tell you that something bad happened medically because that sounds more macho. In truth, what happened was that I had a panic attack. When the doctors first told me that, I couldn't believe what they were telling me. It felt as real as any bout with pneumonia or congested lungs or infection. But they were telling me that it was all in my head. That didn't sound like me at all. I was confused.

In looking back, I realize what had happened to me. I was having a battle between my mind and my body. It was like the World Heavyweight Championships were going on inside me. In one corner, my body, telling me that it felt good, and that I needed to do it and that it didn't matter how I felt about Chelsea or our relationship. In the other corner, my conscience, telling me that it was wrong, that I wasn't in love with Chelsea, and it was wrong

240

because I was still in love with Alex. No wonder I almost passed out.

The "Episode," as it is known around here, effectively put an end to our relationship. After that happened, it shed light on our differences, the problems we faced, and why we should not be together. The bottom line was that, while we liked each other, we never felt in love with each other. Chelsea was uncomfortable with my condition, and that kept her from being totally comfortable with me. And I loved her company, loved doing things together, but hadn't fallen "in love" with her. I realized that, though the relationship was fun, it was a rebound relationship, something to temporarily fulfill my needs. But it could not fill the hole in my heart. That was too big.

We parted soon after that, neither one of us upset or angry. We were mature about it. We knew it wasn't meant to be. And though we weren't a couple after that, we remained friends. Chelsea still calls me up to see how I am doing. I look forward to talking to her and to maintaining our friendship.

The summer came to an uneventful end. For the most part, my days were frittered away, many spent deep in thought and self-analysis. Though I had made two new friends, I hadn't accomplished much else that summer except to gain some new insight into myself. And, quite frankly, it wasn't pretty.

As fall approached, I was headed to college without any plan or motivation. My friends scattered, chasing their dreams and making their way in life, while I sat in Fulton, confused. The only thing that I knew for sure is that I still had deep feelings for Alex. Everything else was uncertain.

As the clock ticked down to my first day of college, I hungered for some certainty in my life.

Chapter Twenty-Seven: Risky Behavior

Toward the end of my senior year of high school, I was forced to make some decisions, just like everyone else that age: what did I want to do with my life? Everyone assumed that I would go to college because I had good grades, but I wasn't so sure. More books. More work. Why? After some arm-twisting I settled on a compromise: I enrolled in a local community college part-time to test the waters.

I set foot on campus without a sliver of excitement inside me. Everyone around me kept talking about the new life or the path ahead. New, new, new. All that I could see was that my life was again going to change. All that I could see was more struggles ahead; and for someone who had to deal with the possibility of dying each and every day of his life, I was aching for something easy, and something fun and exciting. I didn't see that happening any time in the near future.

My college life was off to a bad start even before I set foot in a classroom. I was immediately treated differently from everyone else, and there was no way that I was going to stand for that. For some reason, college officials saw my wheelchair and figured that I hadn't earned my diploma on my own. They never admitted as much. No one ever came right out and accused me of getting help or not doing my work. Still, their message was received loud and clear. They suggested that I take some refresher courses, which in my mind meant that I had to go back to high school all over again. I felt that they were being unfair, either underestimating my abilities, or being prejudiced. So, I flat out refused. There was no way that I was going to repeat something that I had already done.

Then I was asked to select my major. I didn't see the need to pick one right away. Once again, my views differed from college officials. I couldn't see the logic of having to decide your life's path before sampling some of it and exploring some of the possibilities. This idea didn't fly with the college's way of thinking, so I was forced to make a choice. I wasn't excited about anything that I saw in the course catalog. I also couldn't see a reason why I needed to take any classes that did not relate to my major field of study. It seemed so pointless to me, like studying Chinese when you want to be a French teacher, or auto mechanics when you want to be a chef. I could not see any connection at all.

I decided to seek a degree in accounting. It was the least "unappealing" curriculum available. Everything else just looked deadly boring. And after all, I was pretty sharp in math, so how tough could it be? I decided to start college slowly, just to get accustomed to it a little at a time instead of plunging right in. I enrolled as a part-time student, just to see what it was like, taking only two courses, and one of those was to be taken online. That meant that I only had to go to class one day a week to take an introductory business class. Although at the time that appealed to me, what it ultimately did was sabotage any chance I had at putting down roots and feeling connected to the place.

None of my friends attended the school, so that meant starting all over once again and making new friends, if I were to have any friends at all. But this was college and not high school. People were not thrown together for long periods of time. It was not easy to get to know other students, as a lot of them would go to class and then leave for home immediately afterwards. The only familiar face was that of my nurse. Everyone else was a total stranger. The campus was not very conducive to social gatherings and personal interaction. It was just too tiny. That didn't help me to meet people. In no time at all I felt completely alone and isolated from everyone else. I grew increasingly bored as each day passed.

Luckily, my mother had scheduled our family to take another trip to Disney World, which was all set to take place a couple of weeks into the semester. She had been planning this trip for quite a while, setting it for late September. Of course that meant taking a week off from school, but since it meant only missing one class at the college, it was no big deal. By that time, I needed to do something fun, so I welcomed this trip with enthusiasm. It was a pleasure to forget about the books and focus on some mouse ears for a change.

I was very excited to get away; and I was even more excited that we were going to fly down there. I liked flying very much, as a jet was the only thing that could almost keep up with me…almost!

They had to make special arrangements for me when I flew because, by that time, I was traveling with my nurse and an arsenal of equipment. Getting onto the plane was no easy task. I had to be checked in and examined in a special area. Then, all my gear was carefully stowed in the belly of the plane, while someone hand-carried me to my seat and fastened me in place. This, of course, was all supervised by family members and my nurse. Then, for a few brief hours, I was above it all, soaring through the clouds, alone with my thoughts…and a soda and a bag of peanuts.

We arrived in Orlando and made our way to our hotel, The Coronado Springs Resort in Disney World. A fancier place I have never seen in my entire life. The rooms were huge, just like everything else: the lobby, the fountains, and the pool. And the food was out of this world! In no time I forgot all about accounting and numbers, unless it was to count the numbers of burgers that I had devoured that day or the number of pretty girls that had passed by. I was starting to feel like my old self again.

While the hotel was great, Disney World was even better. Cralynne and I were super-excited about this particular trip because my nurse had come with us. That essentially meant we could ditch the rest of the family and wander around on our own. I loved the sense of freedom that it gave me, just to be able to do whatever I wanted to do, whenever I wanted to do it. There were no schedules, no set times to be anyplace. It was just total fun and freedom.

I read a sign in Disney World which said "The Happiest Place on Earth." I thought about that sign a lot while I was there. I thought about it, not just because I was happy there, but because I knew that I wasn't happy other places. I began to wonder why that was true for me, and I figured out why.

In Disney World there were so many things I could do that I couldn't do anyplace else. There were a lot of rides that I could go on while I was still in my wheelchair. In fact, the whole place is welcoming to wheelchair-bound people. It wasn't a case of someone designing an amusement park and leaving it like that. It wasn't even a case of someone building an amusement park and adapting a few things for people in chairs. No, just the opposite. The people who built Disney World wanted to create a place where *everyone* was welcome, where *everyone* was just like everyone else. It was a place where I felt at home.

There is a certain beauty in letting go of everyday worries, of sitting back and becoming a kid again, and feeling the warm sun against your face and the rush of the wind through your hair as you glide effortlessly on your ride. There is a heavenly feel to a place where laughter fills the air, and thoughts of the fragility of life float away to the sky and drift off with the passing clouds. My time in Disney World gave me the chance to escape everything. It was perfect.

Our week in Florida ended much too quickly. Soon it was time to get back to reality. As we gathered our things to make the trip back to the airport, I didn't feel like talking to anyone. I could feel inner tension already starting and a knot starting to tighten in my stomach. On the plane, all I could think was "What now?" I was stuck in a place where I did not want to be, listening to lectures about subjects that bored me to death. I wasn't in a relationship with anyone. And I only had a few friends who were still in town. I felt lost and confused once again. I was headed for trouble fast.

There have been times in my life when I have acted out. There have been times when I have rebelled, acted wildly, or even hurt people. But those times usually stemmed from a single issue in my life that was not going well. But during the fall of 2007, it seemed like *nothing* was going the way that I wanted. I had way too many issues to deal with. I saw no future for the boy who always smiled. As a result, I acted as if I just didn't care at all – because I didn't.

In the fall of 2007, I completely ignored the notion that a person is responsible for their actions. I am not proud of what I did, but hey, I'm normal. I did what any normal, red-blooded male would do when depressed, confused and facing a dark future: I went wild. I acted recklessly, selfishly, and very, very dangerously.

I began ignoring school as much as possible. Oh, I went to class alright, but my mind was far off someplace else. I didn't want to be there. It was as plain as that. I was not in love with the campus. The place gave me the feeling I was trapped. My body itched to break free and escape every minute I spent there.

At home, I was more at ease, but still itching for some kicks. I began doing anything and everything that popped into my head regardless of the consequences, making sure I stayed just shy of getting into trouble. Friends would come over and we'd go outside my room and set up our amplifiers. Then we'd jam with the volume set as loud as it could go; blasting out the neighborhood until 10:00 p.m., the time when the police could be called. We always stayed one step ahead of the cops, so ten o'clock was quitting time for the music, but starting time to cruise around town.

I was spending a lot of time with J.T., Johnny, and a few others who fed into my feelings of rebelliousness, adding fuel to the fire and mischievous thoughts to my head. Most of my buddies were older than me, so they had access to a higher level of "tools" that we could use to get a few laughs. And we took advantage of them whenever we could.

Once in a while, a few of my friends and I would cross the street and climb a small hill directly across from my house. While we were there, safely behind the cover of some trees, we shot off fireworks and filled the air with noise and smoke. These were not the tiny firecrackers that little kids use, either. These were huge and loud and dangerous, just like my life had become. We'd do this whenever we had a chance. Then we'd rush back to my place, just seconds before anyone had a chance to catch us.

Some of my friends smoked cigarettes, so of course that meant being offered to join them. Up until that point, I had always resisted, knowing how deadly they could be in my condition. Those days were over. I began smoking. I didn't care about the risk I was taking: how breathing was already difficult and what filling fragile lungs with smoke could do. I know it sounds insane, but it's the truth. I had no regard for what it could do to me. At that point, I didn't see any future, so I let my friends hold a cigarette in my mouth

248

while I puffed away. Luckily, one of my nurses – who are normally just supposed to keep in the background – got in my face, yelling and threatening me about the dangers of what I was doing. After that, I stopped – and moved to alcohol.

I wanted to see what it felt like to be drunk, and I did. Again I didn't care what the risks or consequences might be; how dangerous it could be for me to become sick and vomit. I put my life – and all that hard work of fighting my illness – in jeopardy.

As everyone commonly knows, trying a cigarette and sampling an adult beverage are, on their own, quite incomplete. In order to complete the time-tested trifecta of wild behavior, you have to throw in one more thing: women. That is exactly what we did.

Johnny and I didn't spend all of our time in my room. Far from it. At that point in my life, as far as the opposite sex was concerned, women were like a Whitman's Sampler. So many different ones out there. I wanted to sample them all.

Most evenings, right around the time when everyone was supposed to be quiet, Johnny and I would leave the house and prowl all over town. It was our version of cruising. Sometimes we'd meet women and hit it off. Sometimes, we would end up with phone numbers. Sometimes the phone numbers led to dates. Sometimes much more. We were very successful. But Johnny and I didn't always roam around town to find women. Sometimes he would show up at my door with two of them in hand. It saved a lot of time that way. After that, my nurse would leave the room to allow us to have as much private time as we needed.

One day, however, everything didn't go off exactly as planned. Although my nurse was carefully standing guard by the entrance to my living area, my grandpa accidentally slipped past her. He bounded into my room and got an eyeful. He got a good glimpse of my date and me having sex. And even though I noticed he was there, there was no way I was going to stop. Startled by what he had seen, he let out a gasp, and quickly retreated into the rest of the house, singing some "Jesus music" at the top of his lungs as he made his swift exit. To this day, my nurse will still bring up the subject and smile. Grandpa never said a word.

The rest of my semester went just like this: show up for class, avoid work, and do stupid things the rest of the time. I managed to pass both of my classes without putting forth much effort, so that kept everyone off my back. And as the holiday season approached, I was exactly where I was when I started college – lost, confused and bored – with the prospect of doubling my workload as a full-time student looming ahead of me. I wasn't looking forward to a thing. Something had to give.

That Christmas was a sad one for me. The weather was bad, as usual, and that left me with a lot of time on my hands to think out how I had been behaving. I realized that I had made a lot of mistakes. I realized that I had been acting badly. I wanted to change, yet I had no motivation to do so. But sometimes, fate has a way of stepping in and doing that for you. It makes you realize what's important. A short while into the next semester, I contracted pneumonia again.

"What next?" I thought, *"Whenever I try to get my act together, I get sick. What's the use?"*

I was disgusted by my circumstances. The prospect of fighting another illness, while missing classes and having my work pile up only made me feel worse. I wanted to be a good student, but this was going to make it tough.

And then I got worse. I was stuck in my bed again. I had a fever and I was struggling to breathe. My mom called 911. I needed to get to the hospital.

"I'm sorry, Craig. You're not getting better. We have to get you to the hospital. I have to call 9-1-1. It's the only way. We have no choice."

Not again, I thought. *Oh God, please. Not again*

My machines stopped working. After that point, all that I remember of that day was the panic. I faded in and out of consciousness until a cold and deep darkness overtook me. I was someplace else, someplace where I had never been before. The doctors said I stopped breathing several times. The doctors said I turned blue. But I was never "officially" told that I had died…but that is what I believe happened. I truly believe that I died that day and then came back. I do not remember seeing a light, as some people say. I only know that I went someplace. Maybe I didn't go far enough. Maybe I was caught in between. Words cannot describe it. That is how strange it felt.

I remember more about what happened after that. I remember being in the hospital for a week, and fighting to get back to reasonably good health. Those memories are reasonably clear. But what I remember the best is what my latest bout to survive had done to change my life forever.

While I was still in the Intensive Care Unit, my mom went down to my college and withdrew me for the semester. As soon as she spoke to the doctors, she knew that there was no way that I could be nursed to health good enough to resume my studies until the next year. When she told me about this, I agreed with her. Also, I felt a great sense of relief. Now I had one less thing to worry about. All that I needed to do was to focus on my health for a while. There was to be no going to school, no worrying about classes or grades, no worrying about my future, and definitely no bad behavior either. In a

251

sense, it was comforting to know what the next few months would be like. Fighting illness was familiar to me, and I like feeling familiar.

While I was recovering, it became clear that I did not want to go back to school. The trick now was to tell everyone about my decision and let the chips fall where they may. I knew it wasn't going to be easy, since Mom placed a lot of importance on education, but I was hoping that her common sense would make her see the light. College wasn't right for me, at least at that point.

Right about the time when I was going to have to break the news to Mom, something happened to make it easier for her to swallow.

"Craig, I have some bad news," she said.

I couldn't imagine what that could be unless it meant that my latest checkup showed a setback. The prospect of that scared me.

"I just got back from the Registrar's Office where I was trying to get information about starting school again next fall and…"

"What is it, Mom?" I asked. "Just say it."

"Well, it seems as if you lost all of your financial aid," Mom explained on the verge of tears. "I am so, so sorry. Maybe we can find a way…"

"Mom," I started. "Don't. I don't want to go back."

"But –"

"It's not for me," I explained.

"But, it's college."

"I know. It's college. It's an education and that is important. But it doesn't feel right. Not now. Not at this point in my life. This is

252

not what I want. I am sure of it. You have to trust me about this. There's something else out there for me. I am positive."

Mom listened carefully to every single word that I said. She did not argue with me because she knew that all the education in the world did not matter if your heart was someplace else. Your heart and your head had to be in it together.

"OK, if you want to do something else with your life, then that's how it should be."

The trick now was to find out what that was.

Chapter Twenty-Eight: Not Again

Finally…relief. By the time the summer of 2008 rolled along, some decisions had been made. I knew what I was going to do with my life – or, more accurately, I knew what I wasn't going to do. I wasn't going back to school. And while that may sound negative, it wasn't. Deciding not to go back to school was the first step on the road to getting my life back in order.

Sometimes life can seem like the first time you walk into a candy store filled to the ceiling with treats of every kind, shape, and flavor. But in this candy store, you don't recognize any of the sweets and you have no idea what they will taste like. You have no idea what you might or might not like. And then the man at the counter asks you what you will have. So, what do you say? It's impossible to make a decision.

That's where I was in 2008; at the entrance to the candy store, looking the shelves up and down, wanting to try something sweet. But I wasn't as lost or confused as the boy who didn't know what he wanted, because I had one advantage: I knew what I *didn't* want: college. After that, everything else was fair game; so it was up to me to pop a few sweets into my mouth and see how they tasted. That was no problem at all. I wanted to sample life to the fullest.

I am happy to say that my family did not put pressure on me to do anything. They were well aware of the challenges that I faced, and they knew the importance of letting a person decide what to do with their life. As a result, they gave me some space. I was allowed to relax, goof off, and do whatever I wanted. They gave me time to sort things out, which is exactly what I needed.

Deep down I knew that this respite, this little break from reality had to end. Sooner or later I would have to try my hand at a career of some sort, and not just sit around all day with my friends, my guitars and my videos games, as appealing as that sounded. Sooner or later I would have to decide what I wanted to be. But at that time, the list seemed like a short one. I always wanted to try hockey, though sports was out, unless they could find a way to get ice skates onto my chair. A pilot? Nope. A firefighter? I don't think so. A brain surgeon? It didn't seem likely. At that point in my life, nothing popped to mind, unless there was an opening in the world of women's cosmetics. If they needed a volunteer to be kissed by women in order to determine if their lipstick smeared or not, you could sign me up immediately.

The only thing that I knew for sure at that point was that the decision was going to depend on what I wanted to do, and not what I could or could not do. I had always figured that if there was something that I wanted to do, and people told me that I couldn't, then I would find a way to do it. I still feel that way.

I was settling into what I saw as a fun time. My room was buzzing with nonstop activity, as my friends were over night and day. I began jamming with a group of guys, casually at first, but more seriously as time passed. I had visions of a band starting; and I started dabbling in songwriting during my alone time. I saw the occasional girl, though relationships had been firmly placed on the back burner. A serious relationship took work and brought the painful possibility of breakup. I wanted none of that, not at that point. I was much more concerned with spending time with my bros than with members of the female persuasion, even though tempted. I was busy, content, and I was beginning to get my optimism back.

Just then, I was plunked right between the eyes with a high, hard fastball. Life was ready to do battle with me once again. Pneumonia, my arch enemy had returned. And this time it was bad.

I was confined to my room, bedridden. The place all of a sudden had become more of a hospital room than someplace where I had fun. Friends could not visit longer than to pop in and see how I was doing. Through bleary eyes I would see a face now and then, mumbling some incoherent words of encouragement while faking a brave smile, the kind people get where you know they are hiding some bad information.

For the first time in my life, doctors had placed me on intravenous tubes, right at home. I was pricked and poked, bruised and sore as I drifted back and forth from long periods of sleep to short bursts of lucid reality. My hospital room was rapidly becoming my prison, and it felt like I was on death row.

My mother, by my side during a lot of my struggle, grew worried.

"Craig, would you like to try and sit up?"

I didn't have the strength to shake my head "no," and I didn't feel like talking. Mom patiently sat there, rubbing her fingers across my brow, trying her best to coax me back to health.

"Why don't you try watching some TV? Or music? How about something you like?"

I couldn't manage a reply. I couldn't focus on anything. The only thought running through my mind was, "This is it." I looked up at my sweet mother, always by my side, always there to support me. I had to tell her something. I owed it to her. Summoning my strength,

I spoke.

"I'm tired."

Mom started to cry. She knew what it meant. Two simple words told her everything. I was tired of fighting the fight. I was ready to give up.

"No, Craig, no," Mom said through her tears. "You're just sick again. That's all. You're just sick and it's draining you. You can't think straight – you shouldn't try to think right now. Just rest up. Just relax and rest."

I didn't say anything more because I *couldn't* say anything more. My strength was gone. My will was fading. All that I could feel was Mom's fingers against my skin as I drifted away again.

The days began to blur – and accumulate. Four, five, six and more. Night and day melted into one long heartbeat, as time didn't seem to matter. A week had passed and I was still ill, tended to by dark, gray faces who popped in and out of focus. I could not move. I could not think. I could not breathe. I was helpless to my fate.

Frail and thin, the medicine eventually began to work. Somewhere around day eight, I started to rebound. People spoke and their words made sense. And even though I still could not reply to them, the dark mood that surrounded me in the room lifted. And then, on day ten, two simple words brought the episode to an end.

"I'm hungry," I said, as smiles responded to my declaration. I was back.

One of the carrots that Mom dangled in front of me to help with my recovery was the promise of another family vacation. This time, Mom promised that if I got better we could all go to the beach – not just any beach, like the small freshwater beaches that we visited on Lake Ontario – but an ocean beach, with real salt water and crashing waves. The thought never left my mind. I became obsessed about it.

"Hey, Mom, when do we leave?" I asked day in and day out.

"Not yet."

"But you promised."

"Yes, I promised we could go after you got better," she explained.

"I'm better! Can't you tell? I'm ready to go. Let's pack the van."

"You're jumping the gun again. You're just a little bit too eager…"

"You promised."

"I know, I know, and we'll go. Just not yet."

"So, when?"

"Let's give it another week or so," she explained. "We have to make sure you are fine. We can't risk a relapse. You wouldn't want that, would you?"

There was no arguing with Mom's logic. What was the point to go to the ocean if you couldn't enjoy it? There was nothing left to do but wait…and annoy everyone by pestering them to death about the trip.

August arrived and I got a clean bill of health – well, as clean a bill of health as I could ever get. That meant we could go on the trip. Mom booked a reservation for a hotel right on the beach at Ocean City, Maryland. Five whole days of fun in the sun, the smell of salt in the air, and the sights of pretty girls walking by, all scantily clad. Sign me up!

As is consistent with the pendulum of my life, the lowest of my lows is often followed by the highest of highs. And that is just what happened during our all-too-brief stay at Ocean City. The trip was just perfect – my best vacation to date – and I loved every minute of it.

This was my first trip to the ocean. I fell in love with it. The entire place was a beach-lover's paradise. Long stretches of sandy beach reached up and down the coast. Gentle waves washed ashore, depositing shells and lifting bathers up and down as they cooled off. The smell of sunscreens of every variety all mingled together so that the air was filled with the fragrant mix of flowers and cocoa butter.

If one got tired of the peaceful beauty of the beach, there was always the excitement of the boardwalk, which stretched as far as the eye could see. There the air was thick with the aroma of every kind of food imaginable, from seafood to burgers to Chinese food. And the shops all blasted heart-thumping techno music to attract the wandering eye.

Pretty girls were everywhere: walking along the beach (usually in pairs), strolling through town, browsing in the stores, and working in the shops. They were everywhere. Naturally I tried to strike up a conversation with more than a few of these girls from time to time. Soon, I began to notice something very interesting, besides the usual things that I noticed. A lot of these girls were from Russia.

There is an old movie called "From Russia with Love" whose title perfectly described my five days in Ocean City. It was like falling in love every 15 minutes. I started feeling like that boy in the candy store needed some sweets, and needed them right away.

There was one girl in particular who caught my eye. Her name was Irina. Irina worked in a shop that sold all kinds of novelties and odds and ends. The merchandise was mostly junk, but that only served to make her stand out even more. Seeing such beauty cast against a sea of novelty items made her glow. Short, dark, and very healthy, Irina was definitely eye-candy. I could not stop looking at her the whole time I was in her store.

The first time there I bought a T-shirt. We chatted a while as I paid for it. I fell in love with her cute accent. As she handed me the bag, she smiled at me, which made it difficult to leave. After that, I made sure that I checked back at least once a day to see if she was working. We talked every time I bought something that I inevitably "needed" each and every day: extra-large sunglasses, a beach towel, a seashell necklace, five shot glasses, and some fake teeth, to name a few.

Our time at Ocean City ended much too soon, but my wallet was looking rather thin; and it was clear that a few more trips to see Irina and I would be broke. Reluctantly, it was time to head back north. I just wish I could have taken her with me.

I wish that I could say that my trip to the ocean and the remainder of the summer served to get my life back on track, but I can't lie. I wasn't over the hump yet. My life back in Fulton settled into a comfortable routine, and that's just what it was: routine. And that wasn't OK because I wanted my life to be special.

Soon, having answers didn't matter, as I was again hit with that big question: live or die? Two months of good health was just about wiped out by yet another bout with pneumonia – this one even more deadly than the last. This duel with pneumonia was more like a tag-team wrestling match, as my arch rival was accompanied by a severe case of bronchitis. Once again the doctors prepared me, informed me, and instructed me. But I already I knew the drill. Once again we were set to do battle at home, since home was actually better-equipped than the hospital. At home, I had all the machines that I needed to keep me alive. I had wonderfully-trained nurses – each one adept at operating the machines and at spotting my needs in the blink of an eye – at my side 24 hours a day. Thorough and competent as a hospital might be, there was no way that they could offer me that kind of attention. The bottom line was that I was safer at home.

But even with all this care, I was losing the fight. This attack of pneumonia was worse than the last. After a week or so, my condition was worsening and the doctors were at a loss as to what to try next. My pulmonologist was running out of ideas and getting worried.

"Starr, I think it's time to make some decisions," he said to my mother.

"Decisions? What does that mean?" she asked. "What's to decide? Is there another medicine that might help? What more can be done?"

"No, Starr, I'm afraid there isn't. I'm afraid there's nothing more we can do."

"Nothing more we can do! There's always something more! I refuse to give up! *We* refuse to give up!"

"I'm not talking about giving up, Starr," he explained.

"Then what are you talking about?"

"There's nothing more we can do here at home. He is getting worse. Craig has to go to the hospital or else…"

There was silence for a second and then he continued.

"Even at the hospital, he might not make it. But at least there's a chance."

"Why? What difference would it make? What can the hospital do that we can't do here? Isn't Craig better off here?"

"No, Starr, I don't believe so. I think that Craig needs to go on a ventilator."

My mother lost it. I have never seen her so angry in my life. To my mom, the word "ventilator" was like a death sentence. It meant never coming off of it. It meant a lifetime of tubes and machines and no freedom. It meant no talking and no singing.

"NO! I refuse! There's no way that my boy is going to be hooked up to one of those! We refused it after the surgery and we will refuse it now! We will find another way. Now get busy and start looking for the answers!"

Mom added a few choice expletives and really unloaded all her fears and anger on the doctor. He grew frustrated and kept trying to convince her to let me go to the hospital. But her mind was made up. It was useless to argue. Time was wasting and we had work to do.

"Very well, Starr, I can't force you to take Craig to the hospital."

"That's right!" Mom said.

"I guess we'll just have to find another way to deal with this."

"And we will!" she added.

After the doctor left, Mom looked me straight in the eyes.

"You're going to get better. Just hang in there a little longer. We'll find the answer."

As far back as I can remember, our philosophy has always been: don't give up, fight back and find answers. We may have tried some unorthodox things – and a few times we didn't listen to the doctors, which maybe wasn't the smart thing, but that was because we have had to be so stubborn and tenacious. When you are dealt such a bad hand, sometimes you have to bluff your opponent…and pray a lot.

When I was little, I heard people talking about something called a "DNR," which is short for "Do Not Resuscitate." I asked my mother what that meant and she told me straight out, just like she always did. I understood that some people get to a point where they are so bad that they chose to let things happen without intervention. It's a personal choice made after conversations between doctor, the patient, his or her family, and after considering the patient's spiritual beliefs.

When Mom told me what DNR meant, I asked her to make sure that they wrote "DNNR" on my charts. I wanted it to say "Do Not NOT Resuscitate." I wanted to take every chance that I had, and explore every possibility out there. There was no way that I was ever going to give up. That's just how I felt.

I think that's why the idea of the ventilator seemed like an ominous specter to us. I know it's not true, but it symbolized giving up. We felt like there would always be something else to try before it came down to that. And so far we have always been right.

The doctor got busy doing research. So did Mom. No one was ready to take that final step until every single possibility was explored. Luckily, as my struggle continued and I was slowly slipping away, there came a breakthrough.

My pulmonologist found out about a new device that had just come out. The device was called a "Frequencer." The Frequencer is like a small defibrillator. It is a tiny machine with a special paddle attached to it, which sends out sound waves. When placed upon the chest the waves vibrate through it and break up secretions that are trapped in the lungs. The Frequencer could be used for hours at a time without stressing the patient. This was a big breakthrough. We decided to give it a try.

We were able to get a Frequencer and have it installed in my room. I was told that I was only the third person ever to try it in the United States. Again I felt very lucky. Soon my treatments began around the clock. It wasn't easy and it wasn't pleasant, but the Frequencer worked, and once again I had beaten pneumonia. My month-long battle came to an end. The Frequencer had saved my life.

I will say it again: I am a very lucky guy. I am lucky to have doctors who keep on top of current developments in the medical field. I am lucky to have both my family and my doctors as a support system that refuses to give up. And I am lucky to have been able to acquire the machines I have needed to keep me alive. I wish everyone could be this lucky. I am truly blessed.

The remainder of 2008 was spent in quiet introspection. A general sense of calm had come over me. It was clear that I had survived some significant trauma in the past six months and I was truly grateful for that. The peace that surrounded my family during the holidays was welcome and we all gave thanks for what we had.

I made up my mind not to worry about my path in life. I decided that it did no good at all to fret about a time frame or a schedule or a plan. I had the feeling that I would know what to do when the time came. It was time for the word "patience" to now enter my vocabulary.

Chapter Twenty-Nine: Music

The winter of 2009 gave way to spring, and as the snow slowly melted away, the whole town began to thaw. So did my frozen life. It was time to stop sitting and thinking and waiting. It was time to do something. But what?

I knew for sure that I was happiest when connecting with other people. The idea of reaching out to others, sharing, and helping appealed to me. I had the urge to express myself and the urge to influence others. To sit alone and isolated seemed wrong. Connecting with others was as natural and necessary to my life as breathing. So, naturally, I turned to the one thing that I thought would do that. I turned to my music.

Although I only had two frustrating guitar lessons, I had nonetheless been able to teach myself how to play, and I was halfway decent at my craft. I had no trouble at all understanding musical concepts and theory. It flowed through me, circulating like the blood in my veins. I was passionate about my guitars and my music, so I felt it was time to spread that passion around.

I came up with the idea of giving guitar lessons. It was no

surprise that when I told my family about it, they were behind me one hundred percent. The next step was to figure out how to launch my career as a music teacher. The first thing we did was to spread the word about what I wanted to do. Everyone felt that this was a good way to test the waters and see if there was any interest out there. By simple word of mouth, I was contacted by a few people. Before you knew it, I had three students.

The easiest thing to do at that point was to give the lessons at my house. Let's face it, whenever I went someplace it was like packing for an African safari. It wasn't as simple as hopping in the van and taking off. I had to be prepared, so a bit of packing and unpacking was always the case. Since I had everything that I needed at home, except the students, I invited them in and we'd see how things went. Things went well.

I scheduled each student for a one-hour session so that they could get personal attention and have plenty of time with their teacher. The schedule worked for me as well, as it also allowed me plenty of free time for me to work on my own music. The notion of performing in a band was still burning inside me.

Life was good during the spring of that year. Soon, I was getting more and more phone calls from people requesting lessons. My business was taking off so much, in fact, that it became too much to handle at the house. There wasn't enough room. I had to look for someplace else where I could teach my students in groups, and not just one at a time.

I found a music studio not too far away. This was the same studio where I took voice lessons as a young boy. They agreed to let me have a place there where I could teach and practice. The only problem was that I had to get there. That's when Grandpa, as reliable as ever, said that it would be his pleasure to drive me there and back whenever needed. I was on my way! I was so excited to have finally found my calling. I looked forward to each and every day with an enthusiasm that I hadn't felt in years.

One ironic thing about my new teaching studio: Remember my initial frustration with the guitar and how I fretted over finding a way to play it? Remember the teacher that told me I would never learn to play, but I did? And now here I was teaching others? Well, next to me at the music studio, teaching his own students how to play, was the teacher I had for those very first two guitar lessons. I guess I fooled him.

As the summer hit, I was busier than ever – maybe busier than I wanted to be. I had eleven students by then and had to turn some away for the lack of time. I was working a solid four days a week, and it was starting to tire me out. I didn't have enough time for my own playing and writing, and the lack of balance started wearing on me.

Another frustration that I had was the occasional student who did not have passion for his instrument. Once in a while, I would get a novice whose parents were forcing him to take an instrument against his will. The guitar is a popular choice, and since everyone fancies themselves a rock star at some point in their life, the kids were directed my way. I didn't have the patience for anyone, no matter what level of skill or talent, who was not serious about learning. My solution was to quickly stress how much hard work went into mastering an instrument. That usually scared away anyone who wasn't at least half as serious as I was about playing the guitar..

Something else equally amazing happened that summer. It was during one of my routine check-ups when it happened. Usually, I didn't pay much attention to what was going on during these things. Most of them were just a long series of medical tests and, if you dwelled upon them, the ordeal could overwhelm or depress you. Most of my time spent in doctor's offices and hospitals was spent

269

daydreaming about beaches filled with pretty girls. But this time, some important results caught my attention.

After a complete battery of tests, the doctor informed us that the results of my Pulmonary Function Test (PFT) puzzled him. At first, I thought he meant that in a bad way. But it was the opposite. According to his results, my pulmonary function was actually improving! This, in his mind, was impossible. I wasn't supposed to improve. I was only supposed to get worse. The results didn't surprise me at all. In my eyes, this was just another case of my doctors underestimating me. I had always planned to get better.

"Maybe now I can keep pneumonia away for good," I thought.

No matter what the reason, the results were good. I firmly intended to settle into a summer filled with good health and lots and lots of music.

And the summer did progress this way. Though not completely satisfied, I felt that I was definitely on the right track. I just had to tweak my plan a little. I just needed more time for my own artistic expression. During the fall of that year, however, the pendulum swung back the other way. After a relatively stable period of time, illness once again found its way into my life. My enemy had returned – only this time I was ready for it.

I was 20 years old, and I had been forced to fight all my life. As a young boy, I didn't think much about what I was doing in terms of fighting. My fight was just instinct. But now I was older and more mature, and I knew what needed to be done. I didn't waste my time doing it. I prepared myself mentally and did not allow negative thoughts to get in my way. From that point forward, whenever pneumonia came my way, I just said "Bring it on." I fight. I get better. I move on. This is my philosophy.

In November of that year, just as I was back to good health again, my sister Cralynne came home one day with a boy on her arm. She introduced him as her boyfriend, Cody, and said she thought we had a lot in common. She wasn't kidding.

"Your sister tells me that you play guitar?" Cody asked, sounding skeptical.

"Yup. It's my passion," I replied.

"But…I mean…"

"How is that possible?" I added, finishing off what he wanted to say, but was just too embarrassed to get the words out of his mouth.

"Yeah, I guess. How can you manage to play? I mean, with your disease and all."

"It wasn't easy," I explained. "I had to come up with my own system."

"Can I see?"

"No problem."

My nurse placed the guitar across my lap, plugged in my amp, but she left the volume in a reasonably-low level. I started playing a few licks, all the while enjoying the look of sheer amazement on Cody's face.

"That is awesome, Bro," he said.

"Thanks," I replied, as humbly as possible.

"Mind if I try?" he asked.

"Do you play?"

"It's my passion," he said. We both chuckled.

"Just grab the other one over there and plug'er in," I said.

It was one of those magical moments that you know in your heart was meant to be. Cody and I were destined to meet. In a nanosecond we became inseparable friends, skipping all of that chit-chat and getting-to-know-you small talk. From that day forward, if anyone wanted to find Cody, they first checked my house.

And Cody and I shared more than a love of music. Cralynne was right; we did have a lot in common. And one of the best things about Cody was that – after that initial awkward moment – he was so comfortable around me. He was at ease with my condition and often did things to help take care of me. It never fazed him one bit.

Soon our casual hanging out and jamming became more and more serious. We listened to music, dissected our favorite songs, memorized chord progressions and our favorite licks, and started developing a sound by adding different distortions to the guitars. It was clear that we were headed toward something exciting, so we decided to take it to the next level. We decided that we needed to form a band. We needed more musicians.

The next person to enter into our circle was a guy named Allen, a friend of Cody's who also played guitar. Then came Thane, Allen's older brother who played bass. The four of us began jamming at my house so that we could get organized. At that point, we essentially had three alternating lead guitarists and a bass player. We needed a drummer to complete the band. I got in touch with Karl, a drummer with whom I used to jam. He agreed to join us. The group was complete.

We needed a name. Every band had a name. Unfortunately, no one was much good at coming up with something that we could all agree upon, so we shelved that idea for a while – at least until we started playing gigs, needed posters, or recorded our first CD.

We needed a place to practice. Four guitars in my room is a little crowded, especially because some of the guitarists liked to jump around a lot. And when you try to fit drums in, too, well, let's just say that breathable air was at a premium. We asked around and were finally given permission to use my church for our makeshift studio, and we started practicing every Monday.

I can still remember the excitement that we all felt the first time we started to play in a big, open room. The fuzzy, distorted power chords rattled the windows, and the reverberated notes echoed through the building. It was a feeling of power and freedom. It was a feeling of musicians coming together and making the whole greater than the sum of its parts. It was a feeling of pure, unadulterated bliss.

If there are any aspiring musicians out there – especially if you are shy, self-taught, and only play in the privacy of your room – I highly recommend joining a band. It is a liberating experience. Not only do you benefit from the knowledge that the other band members bring to the table, you wind up learning a lot about yourself. You learn how to cooperate, share ideas, and blend all kinds of sounds. Most importantly, you will quickly learn if you are any good or not. Trust me on this. The other band members will tell you in a second if you suck or not. It goes with the territory. Emotions, egos and tastes can sometimes clash in a band.

But this was not the case in our still-unnamed band. In fact, we all became great friends. We had similar tastes and were starting to develop our own musical style, greatly influenced by the heavy metal sound. So, even though we were getting along so well, as the summer of 2010 approached, it was surprising to see us having our problems.

273

These problems were not related to anything creative. It was circumstance that did us in. It was the outside world that found its way into our group and forced us apart. It was jobs, education, and the need to earn money to support a family that caused us to dissolve. By the start of summer 2010, our band-without-a-name was officially no more.

Summer was here and I was without a band or a girlfriend. One might think that this would once again be a recipe for another bout with depression. But it wasn't. I had grown so much over the previous year that I was almost impervious to adversity. I was filled with an almost-irrational optimism and I planned to make sure that it lasted a very long time.

I found myself constantly reaching out to others in need. From time to time, people would hear about my amazing medical story and call me up for advice. Sometimes people wanted to know about medicine. Sometimes they wanted to know about doctors or machines. And other times they just needed a boost of optimism, which I was more than happy to share.

I began spending more and more time online as a result of all the emails that I had to answer and messages that I received. I started connecting with numerous people the world over. Sometimes we would seriously correspond; other times we would just chat. And still other times, I would play my video games online against friends old and new. I especially enjoyed playing major league hockey on my X-box. My dream of being in the NHL had come true!

It was then that it dawned upon me. I did not have to teach music to make a difference in the world. I could keep my music as my own personal passion. I would have it forever and no one could take that away from me. Then, if the time or opportunity ever came to share it, I would. But I did not need to base my whole life upon it. I was needed more in other areas.

I also realized that I had a responsibility to share my story with others. I needed to get my information out there in the hopes that others might benefit from some of the blessings that I have had in my life. This would be the best way to help anyone struggling and needing advice. It would be the best way to helps others with this disease, or any disease, or those just struggling with life in general. It came to me as clear as a cloudless sky when your heart tells it that you are in love: Helping others should be my life's calling!

Chapter Thirty: Liar

As word about my longevity spread throughout the medical community, I was being contacted more and more by the families of young people stricken with SMA asking for advice. It became increasingly clear how important comprehensive information about Spinal Muscular Atrophy would be – not only to me, but to many people. And while I tried my best to offer help to those who contacted me, I quickly saw that I had some work to do if I was to do a good job at it. Sure, I had beaten the odds, succeeded beyond expectations, and even improved. I had "lived" my disease; but what did I *really* know about it beyond my immediate experiences? That's when I decided to start doing research.

My goal was to find out as much as I could about Spinal Muscular Atrophy Type 1, analyzing my life and the success of my longevity, combining that with what was known about others with the disease, and then share what I learned. I felt an obligation to share my story and my success with everyone and this is what I wanted to do with my life.

I started looking for information about SMA Type 1 patients, clinical trials, and new medications and treatments. I discovered that there wasn't much to be found and I soon found out why. I learned of a sad word that was applied to my disease. That word was "orphan."

Orphan is a word that is frequently used to describe illnesses, while serious and often deadly, which do not affect enough people to make finding a cure profitable. When I learned this, my heart sank. But the cold, hard statistics could not be denied. While considered "rare," SMA Type 1 was one of the leading causes of infant death. Why? Not because it happened so often, but because everyone who had it, died. Since hardly anyone with SMA Type 1 ever survived the first couple of years of life – and even if they did, they were usually permanently dependent upon machines for food, medication, and breathing – there was no economic reason to help those still alive and struggling. If you happened to make it past age two, you were essentially on your own. You and your doctors would have to improvise treatment, do your own research, and figure out how to stay alive. That was the nature of my disease.

Learning all of this was like slapping me in the face with the biggest challenge of my life – and I never back down from a challenge. If, as doctors suggested, I might be the oldest person (not on a ventilator) to survive with this disease, then it would be up to me to see what I could do to help everyone else who followed in my footsteps. It would be up to me to help all the parents who were devastated when they were confronted with the diagnosis, and every helpless child stamped with this death sentence. It was up to me and I intended to do something about it.

I began contacting every person I came across who had anything to do with SMA and research. Finding the answers I was seeking was like firing a shotgun into the night sky and trying to hit a specific star. The odds were not good. In fact, they were dismal. But then again, what did I care about the odds? Beating them is why I am alive today.

First, I spoke with some research people at the University of North Carolina. Unfortunately, they were only working with people with Duchene's Syndrome and Spinal Muscular Atrophy Type 2. The reason for this was that they could not find any adults who had Type 1. The severity of the disease and the lack of any length of life made finding a cure (or meaningful treatment) difficult, if not impossible.

Then I got in touch with an SMA treatment clinic in Utah, and I was told by doctors there that they had seen some success in treating their young patients with a drug called "albuterol." This was a liquid that could be taken orally several times a day. The doctors told me that, in some cases, it had been shown to build muscle strength or give children a quick burst of energy. It sounded encouraging, so I decided I wanted to give it a try.

When I spoke to my primary care physician, he agreed to prescribe the medication for me, and since then I have taken it three times every day. And though it has not resulted in much muscle improvement, I have seen a great improvement in my overall breathing. It has been a step in the right direction…and I intend to take others.

Since I was so pleased with the results of the advice the clinic in Utah had given me, I immediately called them up and asked if I could travel there so that their doctors could work with me. They told me that there was a doctor in closer driving distance to me who was also doing some remarkable research into SMA. He worked out of Ohio State University and his name was Dr. David Arnold.

Next stop: call Dr. Arnold.

You would think that it would be easy for me to get in to see someone doing research on a disease in which I might be the oldest living person to have it. But that wasn't the case. A few hurdles had to be jumped.

My first phone call was met with doubt and skepticism, to put it mildly. The person on the phone did not believe it when I explained my story to them. They were about to hang up on me, when I pressed the issue. I rattled off a litany of facts about my life as quickly as possible because I was desperate. I could not let this opportunity slip through my fingers. My tenacity worked, and my call was forwarded to another person who worked closely with Dr. Arnold. (Later on it was explained to me that the person who took my call did not believe me because no one with my disease *should* be my age and be able to speak. Everyone else would have died or been on a ventilator. I guess I took them by surprise.)

Finally convinced that I was telling the truth – that I was indeed a 20-year-old survivor of this disease; alive, talking and thriving – the doctors eagerly wanted to get their hands on me. I was given an appointment to meet the staff of doctors in less than two weeks. I was excited! I immediately phoned my mom and told her the good news. Then we made plans for four of us - me, my mom, my stepdad, and my nurse – to make the trip to Ohio. I was off on my journey.

The night before the trip I could not sleep. Thoughts of hope and promise filled my mind, making it impossible to calm down. Luckily, we had to leave early that morning to make the almost eight-hour trip, so that wasn't a problem. I was wide awake and raring to go before everyone else – and I hadn't even had my morning cup of coffee.

We left the house around 5:00 a.m. and headed off. I can still remember the first streaks of daylight and how they lit up the van with a warm, orange glow of optimism. I can remember seeing quick glimpses of Lake Ontario to our right, then Lake Erie as we headed into Ohio.

The day was warm and pleasant as we finally arrived at the vast Ohio State campus. I had never seen anything like it before, almost like a city within a city, beautiful and inviting, and full of hope. We arrived right on time for my appointment with Dr. Arnold and his staff. Before we went in to see them, my mom offered some words of advice, because my eagerness (more like over-enthused, antsy hyperactivity) had been driving everyone crazy.

"Now Craig, I don't want you to put all your eggs in one basket here," she cryptically explained.

"Huh? What does that mean?" I asked.

"It means that I know how you get."

"And what does *that* mean?" I asked again.

"It means that I don't want you to get too excited. This is just a consultation with some doctors. Let's take it one step at a time and see how it goes."

"One step at a time?"

"Look, I don't want you to think that these people will have a cure."

"Why not?"

"Because I don't want you to be upset if they don't."

"I won't," I said, half meaning it and half knowing that it would be again like hearing a death sentence. "I'm not expecting anything, but what's wrong with having hope?"

"Nothing. You should have hope. You should always have hope. I don't want you to ever give up. Ever."

"I won't, Mom. I won't ever," I explained.

And she knew that I meant it.

281

I wish that I could tell you that I met with Dr. Arnold and his staff and that we magically devised a cure in 15 minutes. Of course that didn't happen. I wish that I could tell you that we came up with a long-term plan of attack at that meeting. That was not the case either. Or, I at least wish that I could tell you that it simply went positively. But I can't lie. The meeting did not go well.

Dr. Arnold looked me over. Then several other doctors examined me. I felt a little uncomfortable, like a freak…a science project…something on display. I guess I should have been used to it after all those years, but I wasn't. It still made me uncomfortable, like I was a carcass they were examining, and not a person in the room with them. The doctors talked in a whisper so I could not hear what they were saying. I did not like the looks they were giving me, even though they tried to be pleasant. The doctors talked some more while they went over all the papers that contained my medical history. And then the doctor pulled the rug out from under my whole life.

"Craig, I don't know how to say this," he started.

"What is it?" my mom asked. "Is something wrong, Doctor?"

"No, not at all."

"Then what? Just tell us."

"Well, we've examined Craig and gone over his medical history and…"

By that time my heart was pounding out of my chest. "*What in the world could he have to say*" I kept thinking. "*What in the world?*"

"The fact of the matter is that we don't think Craig has SMA Type 1," Dr. Arnold said. "We think there has been a mistake. We think he has been misdiagnosed."

I was in complete and utter disbelief. I felt like somebody had dipped me into Lake Ontario in wintertime and pulled me out completely encased in ice. My body grew cold and stiff. I felt dead inside.

"No, Doctor, this can't be," Mom said in a slightly raised voice. "Craig has been tested over and over and over."

"Please understand," he clarified. "The facts just do not support the diagnosis. We just don't think that Spinal Muscular Atrophy Type 1 can possibly be what Craig has."

"But, Doctor…"

"Look at him. He sits up in his chair, strong and tall. His breathing is remarkable. He can talk. His functioning is off the charts. There is just no evidence of this diagnosis as being even remotely possible. I am looking at the facts. This cannot be SMA Type 1 here. It must be something else or maybe a less severe type, but that may also be doubtful."

"But, Doctor, he has been tested…"

"There's just one thing left to do," Dr. Arnold explained. "We can confirm the diagnosis with a genetic test. A simple blood test will tell us."

Dr. Arnold gave us the instructions about how to get the blood test. He looked disappointed. I guess he wanted to find the one guy who had survived the longest, and in his eyes, that wasn't me. He was looking at all the cold, hard evidence and it didn't add up. He had to be skeptical because he was a scientist, and scientists need to be one hundred percent sure of things. Only I didn't feel that way. I felt let down. I felt betrayed.

I was completely in shock and unable to speak as they

brought me to get my blood drawn. My whole world had come crashing to the ground with a few, terse words. What next?

A lab attendant greeted me and read the paper that explained what blood test I was supposed to have. He seemed grumpy as he prepared the needle and grabbed a few sterile vials in a matter-of-fact way. Then he tried to find a decent vein with about as much gentleness as a sumo wrestler. I am not sure what he was doing, but as I felt the first poke, I let out a yell.

"Hey! That really hurt!" I exclaimed, which was something I rarely did. I was used to medical procedures and to pain, so for me to speak up, you know it hurt a lot.

"Yeah, oh well," he said as if he didn't care. Then he tried again, digging and poking around under my skin.

If I could have moved my arm, I would have pulled it away. This guy was going at it like a surgeon…only I had not had any anesthesia. He was brutal.

"Hey!" I yelled again. "You think you could find another spot to draw that blood?" I asked.

"Listen," the attendant said to me, "I'm gonna go where I need to go to get your blood."

Stunned by his rudeness, and well aware of my inability to do anything about it, I bit my lip and let him do his job, if that is what you could call it. I watched as he finally hit a vein and then proceeded to drain me of a copious amount of blood.

"What do I care?" I thought. "I don't need it anymore. A lot of good it's doing me. They might as well take it all."

Deep inside my blood was boiling. I saw this as yet another

punch to my gut in an utterly horrible and disappointing day.

My medical experience finally at an end, my entourage made its way to the van and we bolted out of town in shock. No one could think of an optimistic word to say. No one could put a positive spin on what had just happened. It was too new and fresh and completely overwhelming to digest all at once. It was like being forced back to the starting line after almost winning the race. I am sure that the same thought was running through everyone's head: what now?

We got something to eat, but all that I could manage was a few bites. Everyone noticed, but no one spoke. I guess the fretting finally got to Mom because when we got back to the van, she said something. Before we resumed driving, Mom sat beside me, placed her hand on mine, and spoke.

"I know. I know."

That didn't sit well with me.

"What?" I snapped back.

"I know what you're going through, but it's just one setback. Just hang in there like you've always done."

The frustration of hearing those words coming out of the doctor's mouth finally pushed me over the edge. I lost my temper and took it out on everyone; including those I loved the most.

"How do you know what I am going through?" I said in a raised voice. "How does anyone? How does anyone in this family...how does anyone on *earth* know what I am going through?"

"But, Craig –"

"My whole life! My whole life is a lie! Who am I? What am I? What disease do I have? Nothing makes sense anymore."

285

I thought back to all that we had been through over the years; all the struggle and pain. I recalled everyone who sat by my side or lent a hand, helping out to nurse me back to health, or get me the medicine or equipment I needed to stay alive. I thought back to all that we went through to raise money to build the playground, dedicated to a boy with a fatal disease, and now I didn't have that disease. I felt like a crook. I felt like a phony. I felt like a liar. At that moment, I hated who I was.

"What do I tell people? What can I possibly say to explain this? Oh, yeah, right, it was just a little mistake. I don't really have the disease anymore. I never really had it. It was just a misdiagnosis. Just a little glitch."

I was fuming. I could not think straight. I could not see any future. All I could feel was the red hot anger that was boiling over.

"What the hell do I tell people? This is worse than embarrassing. I wish I could crawl into a hole and die! How can I hold my head up around town? I'm a liar. My whole life is a lie. There's nothing left. What the hell do I do now? There's nothing!"

"Craig, slow down!" Mom said trying to calm me. "You're not going to give up. You never will. You'll see. Not now, but soon. Soon, you will be the old C.V. again. Soon we'll all figure out what to do. We always have and we always will. You just can't see it right now. It's too soon."

"And how will I know what to do to get better, when I don't even know what disease I have anymore?" I asked.

"You're forgetting one thing," Mom explained. "There's still that blood test. That blood test could have all the answers. And even if it doesn't, what does it matter? You can still keep working at getting better."

286

I couldn't see it then, but I see it now. Mom was right. What did it matter? Did I need one blood test to define my life? No. Did I need the "official" label of a disease, a name, a title, a word to define who I was? No. No matter what the test said, I had still experienced the same conditions. I had still battled to stay alive against insurmountable odds. This disease – or lack of the disease – was not going to define my life. *I* was going to define it!

We arrived back home sometime between midnight and 1:00 a.m. after a grueling day that lasted almost 20 hours. Exhausted, and still reeling from the experience, we all tried to get some sleep, uncertain of what was to follow.

The next few days were difficult for me. I cut myself off from the rest of the world. I didn't have the words to explain to anyone what had happened, and there was no way that I was going to start unless I absolutely had to. I could not eat. I could not sleep. I did not feel like playing my guitar. All that I could do was sit and wait for that call. There I sat, right by the phone, alone in my room, and waited and waited. Then on Friday the call came.

The doctors were wrong again. The blood tests confirmed it with one hundred percent accuracy. I have Spinal Muscular Atrophy Type 1.

Chapter Thirty-One: Purpose

The day that my diagnosis was confirmed marked the greatest turning point for me, and my life has never, and *will* never, be the same. By the time my twenty-first birthday rolled around, I was a new man.

As far back as I can remember, people have been telling me that I should write my autobiography. To this, I would always chuckle and explain that biographies are meant to be written about famous people: rock stars, actors, and presidents; and I am none of those...yet. Plus, a great many of those people written about are dead, and I wasn't planning on making that journey anytime soon. And while it is true that I have had many interesting and exciting experiences, I wasn't sure if anyone wanted to hear about them. It wasn't until I realized that my experiences might serve to help people that my mind changed. So, as the summer of 2010 drew to an end, I decided to overlook bad experiences and bad feelings because there was no place for ego when it came to helping others.

I told the folks at Ohio State that I would be available to help in any way that I could with their research. If they needed me for interviews, testing or advice, I would be glad to help. And in the meantime, I began composing notes about my life with the goal of turning them into my autobiography.

One of the problems with writing an autobiography – especially when you get to the final chapters – is figuring out how to end it. For a guy who is in his twenties, that can be even more challenging. There really is no good way to wrap it up when you have so much living ahead of you. The story will always end incomplete.

What does the future have in store for me? No one can tell. I could live a hundred years. I could die tomorrow. But I want everyone to know this: never feel sad for me.

Do not pity me or my life. Do not define me by my disease. Judge me as a whole person. If my life is ever cut short, do not shed a tear. Instead rejoice! Rejoice for that little boy who was not supposed to live past three. Rejoice for the young boy who stepped out into the world and touched the lives of others. Rejoice for the young man whose bright smile and angelic voice brought inspiration to people. And rejoice for the man who has loved and lived every minute of his life to the fullest.

ADDENDUM

Reflections on Craig, My Patient, My Friend

Dr. Robert A. Dracker

I first met Craig on January 14, 1994, a little over twenty years ago. At the time, Craig was a four year old child presenting with a one week history of worsening respiratory symptoms. Craig had previously been diagnosed with Werdnig-Hoffman Disease, now termed Spinal Muscle Atrophy, type 1 (SMA-1). Perhaps the most curious aspect of my first encounter with Craig was my appreciation of his precocious, verbally direct nature, especially for such a young child.

Although I was originally warned by the office staff about Craig's conditions and frail respiratory nature, I was not overly concerned since I had early experience with children suffering from malignancies, chronic disabilities and handicaps through my varied training experiences. In fact, I remember that I specifically looked forward to the opportunity to assist him with the healthcare challenges that he would present.

What I soon learned however was that I was clearly naïve and idealistic in my therapeutic pursuit of what would become longstanding medical servitude! Nor could I have been prepared for the unique elements of his herculean strength of mind and his will despite his handicaps, all of which accompany his enduring spirit, endeavoring to survive against all odds and predictions. It was clearly apparent that Craig relished and savored all of the experiences of his life's somewhat restricted reality which many of us tend to overlook and take for granted despite our privileges of self reliance and even ambulation.

Over the past twenty years, Craig and I have overcome repetitive pointless questions, such as "Am I going to die?", or "Are you telling me the truth?" I soon learned that by telling him that yes he was in fact going to die, as I would as well, and that I would try to tell him the truth but if I was lying he would not know it, he finally dropped those questions.

One evening he called me frantically from home, assuring me that he was dying, and he did not think we was going to make it and he needed me to see him right away. I drove from the Syracuse area to his home in Fulton and finally found his house. When I arrived, his mother, grandparents and his home health nurse were all there, and Craig was sitting in his wheelchair, smiling and very happy that I was kind enough to visit him. After allowing him to show me his room, his bass guitar, which he played of course, and then finally getting around to examining him, I informed him that he would in fact live another day and that I was not lying!

Despite the fact that a pediatric neurologist suggested to Craig's parents when he was very young that the only thing they could do for him was to buy him a coffin, Craig lives on, full of life embellished with wit and humor, enduring now for over 24 years. His

292

indomitable spirit lifts and supports me as his physician whenever I see him despite my worst days. Whenever I have the pleasure of his presence in my office, our relationship and discussions deteriorate to those filled with mutual abuse, bantering, love and respect. I have always pledged to be here for Craig as long as he needs me and I have realized that I need Craig to need me in return.

I have told Craig however that there are some limits to what I can allow as his physician. A beer every now and then is acceptable, but no "shots" since it may impair his breathing efforts. He asked me to accompany him and his family on a cruise to make sure he would be okay but I informed him that if I was on a ship with him for any length of time, I would throw myself overboard and then he would have a hard time finding someone to replace me.

Craig cannot and will never stand yet he is taller than most young men I have ever met. Craig has perhaps never had one true love the way many young people his age have experienced, yet very few others have had the benefit of the pure unselfish love that many have for Craig. When Craig quietly whispers to me that he is sometimes afraid of dying, I never tell him how much I fear for my loss of Craig from my life when and IF that day ever comes! I always tell Craig that we all bear "thorns" in our sides but none as deep and as penetrating as he has been in my life. With my love and my care for you always, Dr. Bob.

C.V.'s First Nurse

By Debbie Bernard

C.V. came into my life when he was six months old. For weeks, C.V.'s parents, grandparents, and extended family were almost immobile with grief. Many friends ignored the family, as they were having trouble "dealing" with their own overpowering grief, not knowing what to say and not wanting to get too close. Of course, this caused feelings of resentment and isolation.

Although I didn't know C.V.'s mom and dad, I had known Starr's parents for years, as I had grown up with her oldest sister, Linda. People from our church became involved, providing meals, cleaning the house, and offering as much emotional support as possible. I personally became involved after church one morning in February 1990, when I heard Starr say that neither she nor her mother had slept in three nights. They were afraid that C.V. would choke or stop breathing, so someone was always with him. I'm a "night person" and a "caregiver" (I'm a Registered Nurse and worked the night shift in the local Intensive Care Unit,) so I told the family that I wasn't working that night and would be glad to come to the house so that the family could get some sleep. That night changed my life forever!

The first night I was there, with this beautiful little boy, a report about Muscular Dystrophy was on television. A doctor, who had been doing extensive research in Werdnig-Hoffman Muscular Dystrophy, was talking about how rare this type of dystrophy was and that prenatal testing and treatment modalities were yet to be discovered. I was holding C.V. and crying. I heard Starr come downstairs; I quickly wiped the tears away and changed the channel. She came downstairs about every two hours to check on him the first night I was there. This began a long pattern, lasting three years. My nights off from work, I would spend 10-12 hours at night taking care of C.V., while his family slept.

During those long nights, C.V. and I formed a bond which still continues today. He loved his "kiddy" and "doggy," though he wasn't able to pet them without help. He didn't have to concentrate on physical strides, so his energies went toward his verbal skills. His vocabulary was amazing; everyone thought he was much older. He said "hi" to everyone and was very disappointed if they didn't answer him. He loved going to church and singing in the choir. From the choir loft, I would hear "dink pease," and know he was keeping his mom busy.

One of the best parts of these overnight vigils was the 3 am "parties." Mashed potatoes, pudding, mashed bananas, cake…whatever was in the refrigerator, it was all good. "Mommy" couldn't figure out why he wasn't hungry at breakfast time, until she came downstairs in the middle of one of our "parties." We were caught red-handed. Of course, that didn't stop the parties!

During my nighttime visits, besides doing laundry, dishes, and "quiet" housekeeping, the physical care of C.V. included changing diapers (his mom couldn't figure out how I changed him without waking him up,) turning him at least every two hours to prevent pressure sores from developing, keeping a humidifier running and suction equipment close at hand when he had a respiratory infection, and doing chest PT (physical therapy.) This involved using a cupped hand to rhythmically hit the back while he was in the Trendelenburg position (head down). This helped loosen and drain secretions, and ROM (range of motion), passively moving all of his joints to keep them from getting stiff. He eventually began sleeping in the Trendelenburg position.

Because of his lack of muscle strength he also had trouble burping; when he felt that he needed to burp he would say "bubble" and someone would pick him up to burp him. Whenever I would come into the house C.V. would say "Bebbie bubble," which, of course, meant "pick me up." From then on my name became "Bebbie Bubble." Even now, more than twenty years later, I occasionally hear "Bebbie Bubble."

When the family decided to build a playground and formed the "C.V. Abbot Memorial playground Committee," my nightshift duties changed a little. The entire family and several friends became involved. Once the plans for the fundraising for the playground were formed, I became the "night shift." While C.V. slept, I prepared canisters to go into local businesses, and helped count and prepared weekly updates of the canister totals. I also helped get crafts and food ready for the various fundraisers and managed the bookwork at night as well.

One fundraiser was a concert so I was recruited as the on-sight "medical staff." Most of the day was "medically" quiet; we were almost at the end of the event and I was presented with a guy with a broken jaw. After cleaning the blood from his mouth I gave him an ice-pack. One of his family members was able to drive, so I sent them to the emergency room. I called the ER to give them a heads up. I stopped there on my way home and was told that he had been sent to University Hospital to have his jaw wired.

There was a special "dinosaur" sign made to show the progress of the fundraising. He was called "Parkasorus." My children still have their T-shirts with a Parkasorus on them. When C.V. got tired, during the fundraisers and the building of the playground, I would take him to my house so he could rest where people couldn't find us.

When C.V. was eight months old, the people I worked with arranged for the Easter Bunny to come and visit. We had explained to her that he could not sit on his own and that his legs didn't work. Despite being forewarned she repeatedly tried to stand him on her lap and the floor in front of her. I think that by the end of the visit she finally understood. C.V. loved the entire visit. I'm sure that had nothing to do with the candy he got from the Easter Bunny. He also had visits from Santa, Mrs. Claus and two elves; however, there was no misunderstanding with their visit, as Mrs. Claus was one of the pediatric nurses who occasionally cared for him in the Oswego Hospital.

As C.V. grew, the size and function of his assist devices grew with him. Shortly after he got an electric wheelchair we watched him, in church, turning his chair around in circles. I was standing at the top of the stairs with one of the older ladies of the church when she gave me a strange look and said, "What is he doing? He'll run the battery down." I explained, "He's running!"

Another time at church, after a dinner, someone gave C.V. a broom. He and his electric wheelchair went up and down the room sweeping. People in the room were in awe, but that's how C.V. does things.

At the age of three and a half, C.V.'s doctor decided that he needed round the clock nurses, to not only care for him, but to keep him safe as well. Agency nurses were contracted and continue today. So, at that point I became "just" Aunt Bebbie. I would fill in sometimes, if someone was ill.

"Mischief making" was one of his favorite things. One winter afternoon he was sitting on the floor (the seat of his stroller was removable and he could be set on a base on the floor) playing with his sister Cralynne, when he told her to take his socks off; which she did, although he knew he was supposed to keep them on. Cralynne got yelled at and C.V. said nothing. So the next time he told her to do something for him, she pushed his head back (which he couldn't lift himself) and walked away.

My Buddy

By Mark Bender

My name is Mark Bender. One winter day I came into work at Oswego Hospital where I worked as a respiratory therapist. At shift change the patient work load was split up among the therapists. I have a love for working with children and because of this I always covered the pediatric floor. Little did I know that I was about to meet an amazing little boy that would change my life and I would change his.

I was given a treatment card for Craig Vernon Abbott. I was told by the day shift that Craig, known to all as C.V., was very sick and needed respiratory breathing treatments hourly. Because of C.V.'s medical needs, I was assigned to work with him on an almost one on one basis.

When I first met C.V., I found a two year old blonde haired boy lying on his back in a crib. C.V. suffered from a very rare form of Muscular Dystrophy known as Werdnig Hoffman's Disease. This disease kept him from having the ability to move his legs and limited movement in his hands. What C.V. lacked for muscular control in his limbs, he made up for with his personality and his big brown eyes. No matter where you were, C.V.'s eyes tracked you.

Surrounding C.V. was one of the most loving and supportive families I have ever had the pleasure to know. The only world C.V. knew at this age was the one that his family showed him by carrying

301

him everywhere he went. His world was never by his choice but by the actions of others. His entire life was spent being held or carried.

Day in and day out, my time with C.V. was spent giving him aggressive respiratory care and getting to know an amazing little boy. Over these days, a very special mutual bond and affection grew between C.V. and me. One could not help but love this little boy who made up for his physical shortcoming with his heart.

As C.V.'s hospital stay continued his health progressively declined. The oxygen levels in his blood declined to dangerous levels forcing C.V.'s doctor to try an even more aggressive treatment. It was decided to try ribo viren. This medication is delivered to the patient in a continuous mist form. The patient must be inside a double layered oxygen tent and women of child bearing years were not to have contact with this medication due to its side effects.

C.V. was put into the tents and the medication was started. Because of the double layered tent and the aerosolized medication, C.V. could not see me, or more importantly, his mother and family. Oxygen levels in the tents were kept at levels more than four times the concentration of room air. C.V.'s blood oxygen levels continued to fall and eventually became critical and life threatening. All attempts failed to keep his blood oxygen levels up. It became very clear to me that I was watching a two year old boy die right in front of me. I convinced the pediatric charge nurse to contact C.V.'s doctor, Dr. Kim, and tell her that this treatment was going to kill C.V. Dr. Kim ordered that C.V. immediately be removed from the tents. When he was taken out of the tent, he was almost lifeless and near death. He was placed in his mother's arms with nothing but a simple oxygen mask.

His mother, Starr, rocked C.V. in a dimly lit patient room. Everyone there was certain that his life would slip away in the next minutes.

I was overwhelmed with emotion and I left work early with tears running down my face. I was certain that C.V. had passed in the comfort of his mother's arms with all his family present. The next day I came into work at 3pm as always. My head was hung low and I was struggling to keep my emotions to myself. My locker was in a hall adjacent to the pediatric desk. As I hung my coat up I saw Starr walking up to the nurses' station. I searched for words of condolence without much luck. Oddly enough, Starr seemed happy. When Starr saw me she called to me. Her words were 'There is a little boy here that has been waiting all day to see you." She could tell by the puzzled look on my face that I was confused. She grabbed me and led me down the hall saying "You aren't going to believe this..." Upon reaching C.V.'s room I saw him lying on his back with eyes focused on me. His chest and belly heaved up and down as he called my name repeatedly. He kept asking me if l would play a lengthy list of games with him. Once again a familiar tear ran down my face but was caught by my smile.

As I revisited this miracle on several occasions, I came to believe that C.V.'s change in health was due to his emersion in the love that his family gave him. A few days later, he was released from the hospital to go home.

At the time I was living in an apartment in Fulton, NY. A few days after C.V. was discharged from the hospital I received a telephone call from his mother, Starr. I was surprised to hear from her and asked how C.V. was making out. She told me how he was making good progress, but he continually asked for me. Starr asked if l would be interested in seeing C.V. I was thrilled. I had grown very close to him during his stay at the hospital, but after his discharge I felt I would be crossing the patient - caregiver line to reach out to his family and check in on him.

The next day I stopped over to see C.V. To my surprise, he only lived about a mile and a half from my apartment. We played as we always did during my visit with him. The bond between us was easy to see. After a couple of visits, his mother approached me and asked if Ii would be interested in being a home health care provider for C.V. There had been several issues with finding appropriate nursing care for him. I was working part - time for the hospital and part-time as an Advanced Emergency Medical Technician for Menter Ambulance Service in Fulton.

Although my plate was nearing full, I could not pass up this offer. I met with the nursing company that provided C.V.'s home care. Starr had told them that she wanted me to be one of C.V.'s home aides. After a review of my schooling and credentials, I was told that I was more than trained to save his life, but I had no training to care for him on a daily basis. I agreed to take a home health aide class to get the required "training" and certification to take care of the little boy that had become such an important part of my life. Approximately two weeks later, I was "qualified" to do C.V.'s care.

C.V. lived with his mother, his sister, Cralynne, and his Grandparents, Dick and Molly Wheeler. When I started caring for him, I worked 7 nights a week from 11pm to 7am while the family slept. I also worked numerous other shifts. C.V. had other nurses that cared for him as well, but the relationship he and I had was as friends and not as a caregiver. Even though I tended to his every medical need, C.V. would always ask "Who is my nurse tonight?" When he was told that I was coming, he always replied "I don't have a nurse tonight, just Doogie (a nickname I had adopted working in the hospital)?" Against the nursing agencies regulations, I always wore regular street clothes when I was with C.V. I never felt a 2 year old should have nurses. He should have friends that stayed with him and cared for him. I wanted him to have as normal a life as I could facilitate.

C.V. did not have the ability to roll over, walk, or even crawl. To lift a toy match box car was pushing his limits. Some of my duties were to feed him, bathe him, change his diapers, and move rum where ever he needed to go. Several times a night C.V. would wake and simply say "Doogie, I wanna go on my nudder side." I would reposition him to ensure his comfort. When carrying C.V., you would have to support his head as well as his body. I often carried C.V. in such a way that it would imitate him walking. I would support his chin with one hand while the other ran down his back and supported him under his crotch. With a little rotation back and forth his legs would swing as if he were walking. This became a rather routine way for me to move him around the house. C.V. would often call out to anyone around "Look at me, I'm walking."

When the financial support became available, C.V. was fitted with an electric wheelchair. He was about four years old at this point. This was a life changing time for him. Up until this point C.V. was only moved by others. A wheelchair that responded to him opened up the world for him to explore. When the wheelchair arrived at the house, C.V. spent a couple days trying to work the controls. Starr hovered over C.V. constantly telling him to be careful of this or watch out for that. Her concern for his safety was very evident, but it did not make it easy for this new driver. With a little bit of convincing I talked Starr into taking C.V. to the mall so he could learn to maneuver his new chair in a much more open environment.

With a lot of work we were able to load the chair into the family Suburban and off we went to the mall. When we got to the mall it was no different than it was at home. Starr hovered close to C.V. with her hands near the controls making sure he didn't make a mistake. She continued to tell him to slow down, be careful of this, and watch out for that. I realized it was time for the boys to lose the women and let the little man learn to drive. I used the appeal of clothing stores and the possibility of an amazing sale to pry Starr

305

away from her son. I sent her and Cralynne in one direction and C.V. and I went in the other. Now it was time for boys to be boys. I turned up the speed on C.V.'s chair a bit and released the controls to his eager hand. I walked out in front of him and he soon followed.

The open space was just what this curly haired boy needed. I was amazed at how quickly he mastered the controls. He was thrilled as he rolled down the halls of the mall. He had a smile on his face that went from ear to ear as he called to me "Doogie, look at me...." His smile was contagious to all that saw him. The patrons in the mall stopped and watched this giggling little boy make his way through the crowd. C.V. was just like any other new driver, as he looked from side to side he would steer in the direction his eyes were looking. I will never forget the look on his face when he saw the KB Toy and Hobby shop. He maneuvered his chair into a bee line for the store with his eyes and smile getting bigger the closer he got. After perusing the store, I was able to pry C.V. away. We moved on down the mall where we found the pet store. With precision and grace C.V. moved up and down the aisles of birds, fish, hamsters, kittens and puppies. He could now explore the world he lived in at the speed and direction he chose.

After a few hours of driver's education C.V. was a master at the controls. When we reconnected with his mother and sister I immediately got the death ray look from Starr as she saw us coming down the hall way. C.V. was now running the chair with the speed control all the way up. Starr started to reach for his controls to lower the power level. I grabbed her arm and told her to wait and watch her son. We wondered the mall as she watched in amazement what her little boy had accomplished. A few weeks later I affixed a horn and a siren to C.V.'s chair. It was just what a four year old needed although it might not have been what the adults in the house needed.

As days passed the bond between us grew. I also grew very close to the whole family. Every night when I would get to the Wheeler house there was a huge plate of dinner waiting for me in the refrigerator. The family spoiled me as if I was a blood relation.

I would accompany C.V. on numerous outings. After experiencing C.V.'s disappointment with not being able to do a lot of the things kids his age were doing, I became very determined to minimize this disappointment. I would do everything in my power to let him participate in and enjoy the things that other kids were doing. At a kids play house, I watched kids climbing through a maze of tubes like big gerbils. I turned to Starr and said, "Let's make this happen."

Together we positioned C.V. on my chest as I lay on my back. I pushed and pulled my way around the maze of tubes as C.V. giggled and called to his mother looking down at her through from the portals in the tubes. After this, we moved on to several other games and play structures. When we made our way to a giant pool of balls, I was stopped by the young girl controlling the number of kids allowed in. I told her I had to go in the balls with C.V. She took a look at C.V. and said, "I'm sorry no adults are allowed in here but he can go in by himself." To her defense, looking at C.V. there is nothing physically visible that would lead anyone to believe he was physically challenged. He looked like a cute, curly blonde headed boy with his head resting on my shoulder.

I tried to explain that he was not able to go in alone. She continued to say no. Well, that wasn't working for me. I simply said "Let me explain ...." I picked up C.V.'s hand in the air and let it go. It dropped down to his side without any control or resistance. As a look of understanding and awkwardness came across the girls face a huge smile came across C.V.'s face. Needless to say, he found himself immersed in plastic balls with the rest of the kids. It became a personal quest for me to adapt C.V. or the world around him so he could be like the other kids around him. At one point I built a bowling game for C.V. that had a ramp that sat in his lap. He could hold a plastic ball in his hand and position it where ever he felt was best. When he released it, it would roll down the ramp and strike the plastic bowling pins that sat atop a wooden box. Inside the box I had put strings attached to each pin. By simply pulling a cluster of strings, the pins would pop back up ready for another game.

It was not always fun and games with C.V. Due to his compromised respiratory status, he was often stricken with bronchiolitis or pneumonia. The winter months were always a battle to keep him from getting sick. As part of the effects of the disease, C.V. does not have the ability to have a forceful cough. When sick, mucous would settle into his chest and was virtually impossible to clear. To break up the mucus, C.V. received chest percussion. He would be positioned with his head lower than his hips and someone would "beat" on his back with cupped hands. The sound waves assisted in breaking up the mucus.

At times C.V. would fall asleep in this inverted position exhausted from the fight against the recent sickness. Seeing the benefit of C.V. sleeping in this position, I decided to once again use the wood working skills I inherited from my father. I purchased a crib mattress. I built a frame for it that had the ability to be elevated to different levels. After seeing the benefit of sleeping in this slightly inverted fashion, it was decided by all that this was his new bed. When he was not sick he would sleep at a mild decline and when sick the decline would increase. Because of his inability to roll or move, he never slid off the bed. It was perfect.

I would be amiss if l didn't mention a very special young lady in CV's life. CV's younger sister Cralynne has been an instrumental part of CV's life. Throughout her life, Cralynne has played the role of sister, caregiver, but even more; she is C.V.'s biggest cheerleader.

Often times Cralynne played second fiddle to C.V.'s constant needs.

When I was a senior in high school, my best friend, Jim Sanson, and I had decided that after finishing college we were going to ride our bicycles across the country. In 1992 after caring for C.V. for a couple years, both Jim and I were done with our schooling. It was decided that we were going to carry out our pedal across the USA. C..V's family had always spoken very highly of the make a wish foundation. He had been a wish child just before he had come into my life. Jim and I made the decision to ride across the country, but now we were also going to raise money for the make a wish foundation.

Jim's and my parents jumped in with both feet. In the summer of 1992, Jim and I flew to Seattle Washington and began the trek back to Syracuse, NY. Forty days and 3115 miles later we approached my home town of Fayetteville, NY. We were met by a parade of friends and family escorted by several police and fire trucks. Flying on the side of a fire truck was a banner stating that together we had risen over $4600 for the Make A Wish foundation. Right in the middle of that parade was a curly haired big eyed boy once again smiling from ear to ear. Nearly 20 years later, both Jim's mother and my mother are very actively involved in organizing wishes for terminally ill children in the local area.

Two years later I was accepted into the New York State Police Academy in Albany, NY. Six months later at my graduation as a New York State Trooper there was that same little boy. To this day C.V. and I have continued a friendship and special bond. I cannot explain the honor in being asked by him to write this chapter for his book. C.V. was an amazing boy who has grown into an extraordinary young man against so many odds and obstacles.

Spinal Muscular Atrophy: A Medical Perspective

W. David Arnold, MD

Spinal muscular atrophy (SMA) describes a disorder that causes motor neurons in the spinal cord to function abnormally and sometimes die. Motor neurons are specialized types of nerve cells that control muscles, and when motor neurons do not work, weakness and muscle loss occur. SMA occurs in approximately 1 in every 11,000 births. There are treatments to help with the symptoms of SMA, but there is no known cure. Although SMA is a relatively rare disorder, it is the most common genetic cause of death in infants.

SMA is actually a group of hereditary disorders that affect the motor neurons. Craig was born with the most common form of SMA which is related to deficiency in survival motor neuron (SMN) protein due to a missing or abnormal survival motor neuron 1 (SMN1) gene. This gene problem is responsible for the majority of cases of SMA. Genes are the blueprints inherited from our parents for the many traits and characteristics that make each individual unique. There are two copies for each gene with one copy coming from each parent. Genetic diseases occur because a gene contains missing or abnormal information, and the effects of these changes can lead to missing or abnormal proteins or other consequences that disrupt normal function of body systems. SMA is an autosomal recessive disorder meaning that the disorder will only occur when both copies of the SMN1 gene are missing or abnormal. Most people have two normal copies of the SMN1 gene, but approximately 1 in 50 individuals will have only one normal copy of the SMN1 gene. These individuals will not have symptoms of SMA but are referred to as SMA carriers and may pass on the abnormal gene. If both parents are carriers, the children of these individuals have a one in four chance of developing SMA.

The main symptoms of SMA are related directly or indirectly to muscle weakness and may include difficulty with moving, swallowing, and breathing. Weakness is most noticeable in proximal muscles, the muscles closest to the trunk of the body, and the legs are usually affected more than the arms. The symptoms may be present at birth or may not occur until adulthood. The timing of onset and severity of weakness is related to the type of SMA. There are different ways to classify SMA, but currently SMA is classified into five types based on the severity of weakness and when the symptoms of weakness are first noticed.

The most severe form of SMA is type 0 which causes weakness prior to birth and is fatal shortly after birth without respiratory support. Individuals with SMA type I, also known as Werdnig-Hoffmann disease, are unable to sit independently, and the onset of symptoms is within the first six months of life, often at birth. The majority of patients with SMA have type 1 disease. The symptoms of SMA type II are usually noticed prior to 18 months of age with individuals being able to sit independently but unable to stand or walk. SMA type III, also known as Kugelberg-Welander disease, begins in childhood and independent sitting and standing are achieved. SMA type IV is characterized by onset of symptoms in adulthood. Life expectancy varies with severity. Without breathing support, average lifespan is about 9 months in SMA type I; survival past age 2 is uncommon. Most individuals with SMA II live into adulthood with adequate supportive care. Lifespan is normal in SMA

III and IV.

Craig has experienced weakness from birth and was never been able to walk or sit without support. Based on the onset and severity of his weakness, his SMA is best classified as type I. This classification system is helpful to estimate the course of the disease and prognosis, but it is important to note that occasionally individuals will have features overlapping more than one type of SMA and prognosis will vary. Craig is an excellent example of this fact. In general, SMA type I is considered to have a 0% survival rate past age 20 even with aggressive respiratory support, but Craig has easily surpassed this mark and continues to be able to breathe independently.

The diagnosis of SMA is determined on the combination of characteristic symptoms, physical exam findings, and laboratory testing. The simplest, least invasive, and most accurate way to confirm the diagnosis is genetic testing on a blood sample assessing for the presence or absence (deletion) of the SMN1 gene. With the availability of genetic testing, other diagnostic testing is unnecessary in most cases. If the gene test demonstrates an absence of the SMN1 gene, the diagnosis of SMA is confirmed. In some patients with SMA there is a deletion of one copy of the SMN1 gene and a mutation in the other copy. In such cases more specialized testing with gene sequencing is necessary. Other testing may be considered when genetic testing (including both deletion and mutation of the SMN1 gene) does not confirm the diagnosis.

Prior to the availability of the genetic test in 1995, diagnosis relied on electromyography (EMG) and nerve conduction studies and muscle biopsy. These tests are now mainly used when the diagnosis remains uncertain after genetic testing. EMG involves using a small needle electrode and recording the electrical activity of muscles. Nerve conduction studies involve stimulating nerves with small electrical shocks to measure how the nerves are functioning. EMG and nerve conduction studies can help determine if a nerve or muscle problem is causing the symptoms in question. A muscle biopsy involves removing small pieces of muscle tissue which are then examined for changes suggestive of a muscle or nerve problem.

Craig was diagnosed prior to the existence of genetic testing for SMA. He underwent a muscle biopsy which showed findings supportive of the diagnosis of SMA. Later in 2010 he was evaluated and underwent genetic testing confirming that his diagnosis of SMA was related to the deletion or absence of both copies of the SMN1 gene.

Until an effective treatment or cure becomes available, the management of SMA is centered on treating the symptoms related to muscle weakness. With the help of supportive, care individuals are able to live longer with a higher quality of life. Symptomatic treatment strategies should be individualized to the level of function of the individual. One of the most serious effects of SMA is weakness of the breathing muscles. If the respiratory muscles are weak air cannot be adequately moved in and out of the body. Respiratory muscles also help produce coughing. If coughing is weak, there is an increased risk of lung infections. Respiratory-related problems are a major cause of death in the more severe forms of the disease. Supportive care may include assistive technologies such as non-invasive and invasive ventilatory support and cough assist devices.

Swallowing can be a problem in some individuals. Swallowing weakness can make eating and drinking difficult and may increase the risk of chocking on foods and liquids. If swallowing problems are severe, a feeding tube through the nose or abdominal wall may be used to deliver nutrients to help with feeding and reduce the risk of pneumonia. Mobility and positioning may be significantly impacted in individuals with muscle weakness. Assistive equipment such as power wheelchairs, orthotic devices and bracing, and adaptive equipment can help improve function and independence.

While there are currently no effective treatments in SMA much work is being performed in this area. The level of SMN protein is reduced in SMA due the absence of a functioning SMN1 gene. For reasons that are not entirely clear, when SMN protein is reduced the motor neurons do not function correctly. An additional gene, the survival motor neuron 2 or SMN2 gene, plays a role in determining the severity of SMA. The SMN2 gene also produces SMN protein, although significantly less efficiently compared with SMN1. This gene may partially "rescue" motor neurons. All individuals with SMA have at least one or two copies of the SMN2 gene. Having less than one copy is incompatible with life, and death occurs in utero.

On the other hand, if an individual has additional copies SMN2 the symptoms of SMA are typically less severe. In Craig's case, he has three copies of SMN2. This at least partly explains Craig's remarkably preserved health despite his clinical diagnosis of SMA type I. Strategies have been employed to try to increase the level of SMN protein produced by the SMN2 gene. To date there have been no effective treatments in humans employing this potential mechanism, but this remains a favorable target. Antisense oligonucleotide (ASO) or small molecular therapies are being developed and tested to increase SMN protein from retained copies of the backup SMN2 gene. ASO treatments are currently being tested for safety in early clinical trials. Gene therapy is also a very promising potential treatment strategy. In 2010/2011 several groups showed dramatic rescue of SMA mice treated with gene therapy to replace the SMN1 gene. Without treatment the SMA mice had an average lifespan of approximately 15 days, but after gene therapy, initiated shortly after birth, lifespan was increased beyond 250 days. These findings are extremely exciting, but care should be taken when interpreting these results. Animal models of human disease are created to be as similar as possible, but results are sometimes significantly different in follow up human studies.

Currently plans are moving forward to test gene therapy in infants with type 1 SMA. Cellular replacement of motor neurons using stem cells is another potential therapeutic strategy that is in the very early stages of development. Other potential treatments include treatments to improve the functioning of remaining motor neurons such as neuroprotective agents that help the remaining motor neurons be resistant to further damage. Overall, the field of SMA is experiencing encouraging progress in the understanding SMA and development of promising therapeutic strategies, but continued work is very much needed to take these therapies to the clinic.

ABOUT THE AUTHORS

Craig Vernon Abbott II

Craig V. Abbott II ("C.V.") was born in Upstate New York in 1989. By the time he was six months old, his parents were told that he had Spinal Muscular Atrophy Type 1, a death sentence that was supposed to take his life by age two.

C.V. did more than survive – he triumphed. Despite frequent bouts with pneumonia that nearly claimed him several times, and dozens, if not hundreds of obstacles that were placed in his path, he has gone on to lead a normal life.

C.V. attended school along with his peers, graduating right on schedule. He shared the gift of his angelic voice with others, performing at church and school functions, and singing the national anthem at Syracuse baseball games. When told that he would never be able to play the guitar, he invented his own method of tuning it and playing it. He even went on to become a music instructor and perform in a rock band.

Now a grown man, C.V. is following his calling – to share his story with others and become a motivational speaker. He hopes to instill his "never give up" attitude in others.

Joseph Vincent Abbate, Jr.

Born in New York City during the Mantle-Maris Era, Joe traveled to Upstate New York to attend college, and because he heard rumors that they had snow there. He had no idea what he was getting into.

In college, he met his eventual wife, and they settled in the area because they were still snowed in.

Several years later, Joe was given his own death sentence, when he came down with cancer and was estimated to have between 2 and 5 years to live. He recently celebrated becoming a 27-year cancer survivor.

Since that time, Joe has held several jobs, none more important than that of being a stay-at-home dad and raising his young daughter. He has done a lot of volunteer work in the community, and has worked with at-risk youth, mentoring them in reading and other academic endeavors.

Today, Joe works as a freelance writer, web designer, graphic artist and photographer. Together with C.V., Joe hopes to spread their message of hope and encouragement to anyone struggling with life's problems.